*Molecular Nutrition and Genomics*

## THE WILEY BICENTENNIAL—KNOWLEDGE FOR GENERATIONS

Each generation has its unique needs and aspirations. When Charles Wiley first opened his small printing shop in lower Manhattan in 1807, it was a generation of boundless potential searching for an identity. And we were there, helping to define a new American literary tradition. Over half a century later, in the midst of the Second Industrial Revolution, it was a generation focused on building the future. Once again, we were there, supplying the critical scientific, technical, and engineering knowledge that helped frame the world. Throughout the 20th Century, and into the new millennium, nations began to reach out beyond their own borders and a new international community was born. Wiley was there, expanding its operations around the world to enable a global exchange of ideas, opinions, and know-how.

For 200 years, Wiley has been an integral part of each generation's journey, enabling the flow of information and understanding necessary to meet their needs and fulfill their aspirations. Today, bold new technologies are changing the way we live and learn. Wiley will be there, providing you the must-have knowledge you need to imagine new worlds, new possibilities, and new opportunities.

Generations come and go, but you can always count on Wiley to provide you the knowledge you need, when and where you need it!

**WILLIAM J. PESCE**
PRESIDENT AND CHIEF EXECUTIVE OFFICER

**PETER BOOTH WILEY**
CHAIRMAN OF THE BOARD

# Molecular Nutrition and Genomics

## Nutrition and the Ascent of Humankind

**Mark Lucock**
**BSc(Hons), PhD, MRCPath, CBiol, FIBiol**
University of Newcastle (Australia)
School of Environmental and Life Sciences

**WILEY-LISS**
**A JOHN WILEY & SONS, INC., PUBLICATION**

For general information on our other products and services or for technical support, please contact our Customer
Care Department within the United States at (800) 762-2974, outside the United States at (317) 572-3993 or fax
(317) 572-4002.

Wiley also publishes its books in a variety of electronic formats. Some content that appears in print may not be
available in electronic format. For more information about Wiley products, visit our web site at www.wiley.com.

Wiley Bicentennial Logo: Richard J. Pacifico

*Library of Congress Cataloging-in-Publication Data*

Lucock, Mark.
    Molecular nutrition and genomics : nutrition and the ascent of humankind /
    Mark Lucock.
        p.   cm.
    Includes bibliographical references and index.
    ISBN 978-0-470-08159-4
    1. Nutrition – Genetic aspects.   2. Human evolution.   I. Title.
    QP144.G45L83 2006
    612.3 – dc22                                                    2006052156

Printed in the United States of America

10   9   8   7   6   5   4   3   2   1

*In memory of Anna Martha Marie and John David Lucock*

*This book is dedicated to Rebecca and all students of the life sciences with open and questioning minds*

# Contents

# *Preface*

As a research scientist in the area of human nutrition, I have observed a sea change in emphasis within my field over the past 10–15 years. There have always been dynamics within the subject: During the first half of the twentieth century, scientists grappled with discovering the essential micronutrients and with characterizing the biological effects of their deficiency. This interest in "too little" was supplanted in the mid-1980s by a preoccupation with too much—too much fat, too much sugar, and too much obesity. Unfortunately, nutritional research that looks at the relationship between dietary components and disease has often been dogged by equivocal, even contradictory research publications, frequently undermining the faith that the public has in nutritional science. The advent in recent times of molecular biological approaches to problem solving has moved nutrition away from its origins into the front line of genomic research. Nutrients and genes conspire to modify disease risk, they interact to promote cellular function, and given the variable exogenous disposition of nutrients, have provided a force for evolutionary selection pressures that have led to the emergence of modern man.

Modern nutritional texts have had to adapt to the bioinformatics revolution. Students at the undergraduate and the postgraduate level have had to rethink their ideas of human nutrition. When I began research in the late 1980s, one would typically measure vitamin X in population A and population B and do a statistical comparison to see whether a real difference existed. The research emphasis then changed in the 1990s to see whether variant genes could modify the level of vitamin X and account for the difference between populations A and B. Today we are interested in how vitamins A to Z influence the genome and thousands of gene products in a multidimensional view of cellular processes that we now refer to as nutrigenomics. This is the dawn of the age of molecular nutrition.

Molecular nutrition is a far more multidisciplinary subject than the nutritional sciences of old. It can address fundamental questions of human health that provide exquisite mechanistic explanations of cause and effect. Human nutritional health is an area that I both teach and research, but molecular nutrition can go further than having an impact on health alone. In some ways, given the importance of food components as environmental factors driving evolutionary processes, molecular nutrition may well help explain our human origins. Many groups around the world are now starting to investigate nutrition in the context of human evolution, and in so doing, they are placing my subject within a sphere of endeavor that may well help to explain the meaning of life itself.

I have written this book to help students and teachers at the university level gain a new perspective on an old subject. I have written it in a way that I hope engages students drawn from a range of relevant disciplines that extend from molecular nutrition, nutritional sciences, and nutrition and dietetics to anthropology.

## ACKNOWLEDGMENTS

Given the challenging workload of today's university academic, and the time demands of writing a book, I could never have balanced all sides of my day without the constant support of my family, and so I acknowledge both my wife Jill and daughter Rebecca who continue to keep me buoyant in my personal and professional life, and who pick up the pieces when the pressure gets too much.

It has been my privilege to work with many kind, generous and able scientists over the years. Their encouragement and objective criticism have helped me develop my own perspective on the subject of molecular nutrition, and I hope I can continue a long and prosperous relationship with many of them. I would like to single out Dr. Robert Leeming as a particularly important mentor in my career path.

I'm fortunate to work within a friendly and supportive structure at the University of Newcastle, with many of my immediate colleagues sharing at least some of my research interests. The interactions I have with these colleagues and my postgraduate and myriad undergraduate human nutrition students help me to develop and focus ideas – I value these interactions greatly, not least in terms of the interesting opinions and views on current trends within my discipline area that often emerge. I thank all my former students, present students, and colleagues who are simply too numerous to mention. Each one of you has contributed in some small way to this literary synthesis.

# Introduction

Humankind diverged from our closest primate relatives a mere 7–6 million years ago (1). Even more recently, in fact, a few moments ago by the geological time scale, a revolution in human development occurred; 35,000 to 45,000 years ago, during the Upper Paleolithic era, humans began to create elaborate tools and lengthy routes of supply for raw materials, and they constructed complex shelters and exhibited profound forms of symbolic expression. During this era, higher order behavior appeared across the planet in Europe, North Africa, Asia, and Australia. Since then, it has been an astonishingly short journey to our modern achievements in cosmology and molecular biology at the extremes of scientific endeavor in the twenty-first century. Arguably, no question is of greater interest than learning precisely how we evolved. This book attempts to examine one crucial facet of the huge array of genetic and environmental influences that have forged humankind's recent evolution, namely "how chemical nutrients and genetics have, and indeed still are, conspiring to shape our species".

The complexity that is inherent in postgenomic understanding has led to several new disciplines, for example, in "nutrigenomics" (2) and "sociogenomics" (3) which aim to help define what humankind is at the most fundamental level. Nutrigenomics refers to the interface between environmental nutrients and cellular/genetic processes, whereas sociogenomics blends genomics with neuroscience, behavioral biology, and evolutionary biology. Other disciplines such as "pharmacogenomics" and "toxicogenomics" are highly applied in their goals of searching for improved therapeutic interventions. From recent research in these and related disciplines, it is possible to build up a picture of at least some dynamics that drove our recent evolution at a molecular nutritional level.

The principle is simple enough. Combine natural selection for reproductive advantage with genetic drift, which leads to random changes in gene frequencies. Throw in some genetic mutation, and you have all the ingredients to drive the evolutionary process. To give an example of genetic drift: If two human populations become isolated one from another, random change over time leads to genetically distinct populations. Divergence occurs faster in small populations compared with large ones. Genetic drift within a small population that grows in number is commonly referred to as the "founder effect." The broad picture viewed from a neo-Darwinian perspective is well understood, and is expanded upon later, but how can we explain evolutionary change at the molecular level based on nutrient availability? Is it possible to concoct a recipe for Adam and Eve?

Chapter *1*

# Defining Important Concepts

## 1.1 KEY CONCEPTS IN MOLECULAR BIOLOGY FOR THE STUDY OF HUMAN NUTRITION

Until very recently, the study of human nutrition and molecular biology were considered to be mutually exclusive domains within the biological sciences. This is simply no longer the case. Today, the leading edge of our endeavor to explain the very nature of mankind, and our ascent to planetary dominance blends both nutrition and molecular biology into the fields of nutritional genetics and nutrigenomics. These new disciplines exploit our knowledge of the human genome and its variability to explain how nutrients, their dependent proteins, and encoding genes conspire to forge and maintain our species. These interactions not only help explain the etiology of many diseases, but also they provide a framework for gaining a better understanding of the likely evolution of our species. Human evolution was forged out of our ancestors obligate need to forage for chemical nutrients that varied in their abundance according to habitat and season. This forced early humans to find and compete for limited resources; humans that foraged optimally and competed most successfully for those resources were fitter and more able to reproduce and, hence, could pass on their genetic material to their progeny. In other words, they were selected for. This process of evolution is characterized by a change in gene frequency over time, but what are genes, and how do they lead to the expression of traits, the summation of which produces the state of "being human?" To understand this process, we need to examine the building blocks of our genetic code.

### 1.1.1 Molecular Structure of DNA

Polymeric DNA is composed of four different nucleotides. Each nucleotide consists of a $2'$-deoxyribose sugar, purine or pyrimidine base, and phosphate moiety. Purine bases are either adenine or guanine, whereas pyrimidine bases are either thymine or cytosine. When a base is linked to the $1'$ carbon of the deoxyribose sugar, it is referred to as a nucleoside.

*Molecular Nutrition and Genomics: Nutrition and the Ascent of Humankind*, by Mark Lucock
Copyright © 2007 John Wiley & Sons, Inc.

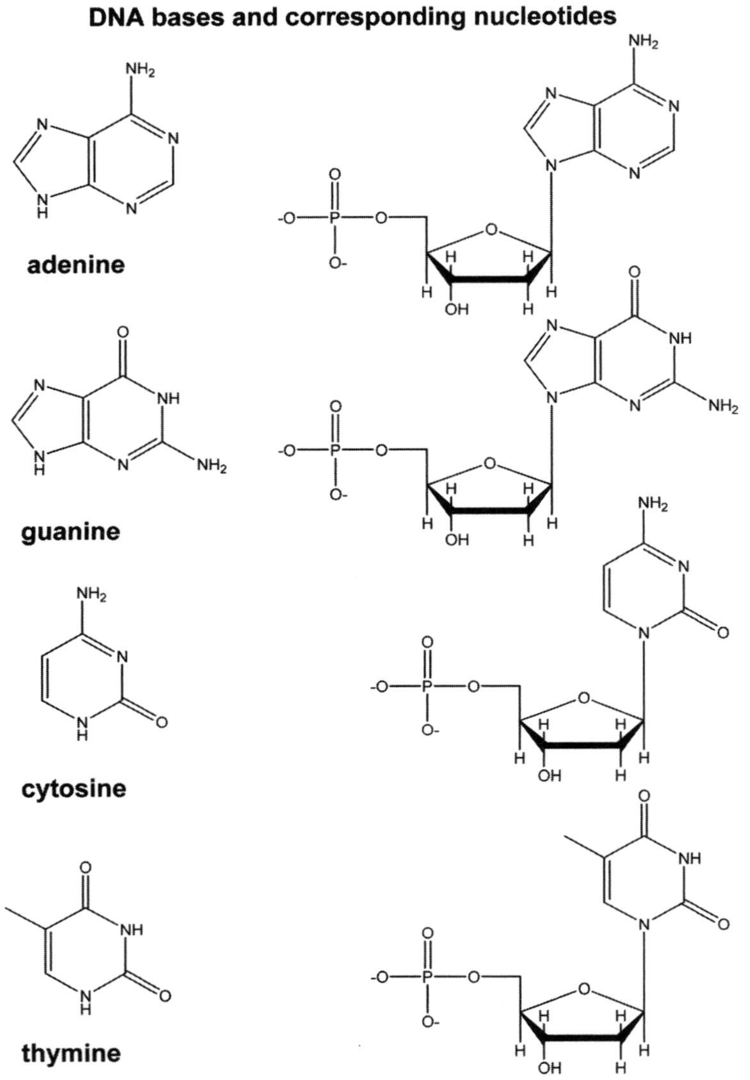

## DNA bases and corresponding nucleotides

**Figure 1.1.** *Bases adenine, guanine, cytosine, and thymine along with their corresponding nucleotides that form the building blocks of DNA.*

When, in addition, phosphate moieties are attached to the sugar, the structure is referred to as a nucleotide.

Nucleotide triphosphates (Figure 1.1) of adenine (A), guanine (G), cytosine (C), and thymine (T) are polymerized to form DNA via phosphodiester bond formation between the 5′ phosphate of one nucleotide and the 3′ hydroxyl group of the next nucleotide. The sequence of bases is what encodes the genetic blueprint for life. It can be read in the 5′ → 3′ or the 3′ → 5′ direction.

The primary sequence of DNA permits a three-dimensional structure to form, which is represented by a double helix. The sugar–phosphate linkage forms the molecular backbone

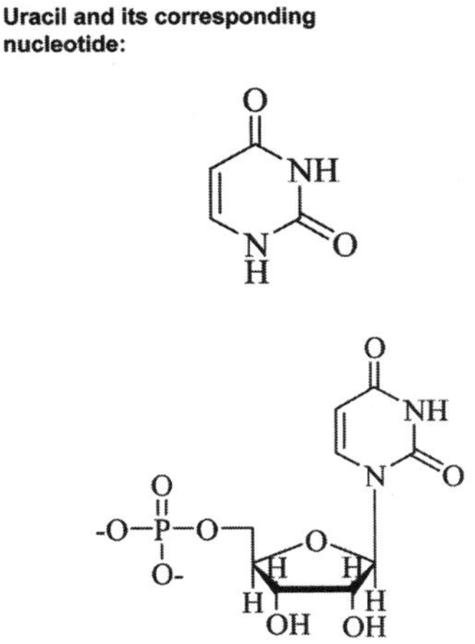

**Uracil and its corresponding nucleotide:**

**Figure 1.2.** *RNA is the same as DNA except RNA contains uracil, whereas DNA contains thymine. Additionally, in RNA, ribose replaces DNA's 2-deoxyribose.*

of this structure. The bases face inward and stabilize the double helix via hydrogen bonds between adjacent T and A bases, and again between adjacent G and C bases. This base pairing is specific, and purine always interacts with pyrimidine, a phenomenon referred to as "complementary base pairing." The double helix is right-handed with a turn every 10 bases. Examination of the structure reveals a major molecular groove, which facilitates protein interactions.

Complimentary base pairing ensures that the sequence of one DNA strand predicts the base sequence of the other. This simple fact is what permits the fidelity of the genetic blueprint to be preserved during replication of DNA as part of cell division, and during the expression of genes.

Expression of DNA, which is the conversion of the base sequence blueprint into an amino acid sequence within a functional protein, requires as a first step, the transcription of the DNA sequence into an RNA transcript. RNA is the same as DNA except RNA contains uracil, whereas DNA contains thymine (Figure 1.2). Additionally, in RNA, ribose replaces DNA's 2-deoxyribose. The RNA transcript is referred to as messenger RNA (mRNA). mRNA is then translated into a protein on the ribosome—transfer RNAs (tRNA) are small molecules that coordinate individual amino acids to form proteins that have been specified by the mRNA sequence.

This phenomenon of gene expression in which the biological data encoded by a gene is made available in terms of a functional protein is referred to as "the central dogma." That is, information is passed from DNA to RNA to protein.

Humans contain around 23,000 genes on 23 chromosomes. These genes are separated by intergenic (noncoding) DNA. Although a gene is the fundamental unit of information in that a single gene codes for a single polypeptide, higher organisms such as man also have multigene families. In their simplest form, a gene family contains more than one copy of a gene where its expression product is required in large amounts. Complex multigene families also exist. These yield similar, but distinct, proteins with related function, for example, the globin polypeptides.

To orchestrate gene regulation according to cellular need, gene promoter regions exist upstream from the coding region of a gene. Promoter sites bind the enzyme for synthesizing the RNA transcript (RNA polymerase II) and any associated transcription factors that are required to initiate mRNA synthesis. Promoter regions usually contain a TATA box around 25 base pairs upstream from the site at which transcription commences. Transcription factors bind DNA around the TATA box and orchestrate the binding of RNA polymerase II. RNA polymerases I and III are associated with transcription of ribosomal RNAs and genes encoding tRNAs, respectively.

Transcription factors can be considered as modular molecules that contain DNA binding, dimerization, and transactivation modalities. These regulatory factors exhibit characteristic structural motifs. The DNA binding modality contains three potential motifs: zinc fingers, basic domains, and helix-turn-helix motifs. Dimerization modalities contain two motifs: leucine zippers and helix-loop-helix structural motifs. The formation of homo- and heterodimers leads to transcription factor variation and, hence, a diversity of function. Transcription factors can act to both initiate and repress transcription.

Genes do not contain a continuous code; rather they are split into coding regions known as exons and noncoding regions known as introns. Introns are removed from the RNA transcript by a process referred to as splicing. This process occurs before protein synthesis.

Some genes have accumulated nonsense errors in their base sequence and no longer function. These archaic genes are referred to as pseudogenes.

### 1.1.2   Molecular Encryption

The base sequence of DNA encodes the amino acid sequence of a polypeptide via the intermediate polymer—RNA. Amino acids are encrypted by 64 triplets; each triplet represents a sequence of three DNA bases and is known as a codon. Within a gene, each set of codons that builds up to form a genetic unit of information is referred to as a reading frame. The reading frame is determined by "initiation" and "stop" codons. In between these initiation and stop codons, one has what is referred to as an "open reading frame."

As the four nucleic acid bases can combine to form 64 permutations of codon (Table 1.1), but only 20 amino acids exist in proteins, all amino acids save tryptophan and methionine are encrypted by more than one codon. This fact is why the genetic code is often referred to as having built-in degeneracy or redundancy. Sixty-one codons encode amino acids, and three are used to terminate protein synthesis (UAA, UGA, UAG). The codon for methionine (AUG) encodes initiation of protein expression. Clearly, all nascent polypeptides therefore start with methionine.

### 1.1.3   Organizing the Human Genome

DNA is organized into cellular structures called chromosomes that are only visible after they have replicated during the cell cycle. Unique structures found at the end of the chromosome are known as telomeres. Telomeres consist of short repetitive DNA sequences. What is of interest in regard to telomeres is the fact that the number of repeat sequences declines with age in somatic cells, but in cancer and germ cells, the enzyme telomerase maintains telomere length (see later). Telomeres are purposeful as they prevent recombination of the chromosomes.

**Table 1.1. Matrix showing how amino acids are encrypted by specific three base codons within RNA.**

| | Amino acid/signal encrypted by codon—the genetic code | | | | |
|---|---|---|---|---|---|
| Initial base at 5′ end | Middle base | | | | Third base at 3′ end |
| | U | C | A | G | |
| U | Phe UUU | Ser UCU | Tyr UAU | Cys UGU | U |
| U | Phe UUC | Ser UCC | Tyr UAC | Cys UGC | C |
| U | Leu UUA | Ser UCA | Stop UAA | Stop UGA | A |
| U | Leu UUG | Ser UCG | Stop UAG | Trp UGG | G |
| C | Leu CUU | Pro CCU | His CAU | Arg CGU | U |
| C | Leu CUC | Pro CCC | His CAC | Arg CGC | C |
| C | Leu CUA | Pro CCA | Gln CAA | Arg CGA | A |
| C | Leu CUG | Pro CCG | Gln CAG | Arg CGG | G |
| A | Ile AUU | Thr ACU | Asn AAU | Ser AGU | U |
| A | Ile AUC | Thr ACC | Asn AAC | Ser AGC | C |
| A | Ile AUA | Thr ACA | Lys AAA | Arg AGA | A |
| A | Met AUG | Thr ACG | Lys AAG | Arg AGG | G |
| G | Val GUU | Ala GCU | Asp GAU | Gly GGU | U |
| G | Val GUC | Ala GCC | Asp GAC | Gly GGC | C |
| G | Val GUA | Ala GCA | Glu GAA | Gly GGA | A |
| G | Val GUG | Ala GCG | Glu GAG | Gly GGG | G |

Chromosomes are actually an aggregation of proteins and DNA. This material is referred to as chromatin. Chromatin that is inactive is known as heterochromatin, whereas active chromatin that permits RNA transcription is known as euchromatin (Figure 1.3). Human gametes are haploid and contain 23 chromosomes, whereas non-sex cells (somatic cells) are diploid and contain 46 chromosomes.

It has been estimated that the entire human genome comprises around 3 billion base pairs. However, the 23,000 human genes account for only a fraction of our entire cellular DNA—the rest is extragenic or "junk" DNA.

As part of the cell cycle, the cell will divide. This entails that chromosomes are replicated. The DNA is copied in the $5' \rightarrow 3'$ direction by the enzyme DNA polymerase using single-stranded DNA as a template.

### 1.1.4 DNA Variation: The Provision of Biological Diversity

Errors in the fidelity of DNA replication along with physical and chemical agents all potentially induce mutations in the DNA sequence. If they affect coding sequences, this may influence the function of any expressed protein. That is, the "phenotype" may alter. The types of mutation include missense, nonsense, and frameshift mutations. All are classified as point mutations. The latter two point mutations have the most serious consequences for the expressed proteins function.

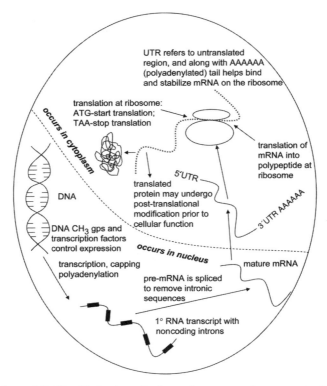

**Figure 1.3.** *Simplified schematic shows the process of gene expression.*

As living organisms are exposed to so many mutagens, life has evolved elaborate DNA repair mechanisms as a counter-measure. The mechanisms include excision-, direct-, and mismatch repair, and they are discussed at length later. This is one area where as an example, antioxidant nutrients prove useful, although they are only one form of defense in this cellular war that is continuously waged within every one of us.

Not all mutations are necessarily bad. A gene that has, for example, an A where previously there was a G, may, under the influence of evolution, become more frequent in successive generations. That is, it is advantageous to possess this mutation in a given environment because it improves reproductive efficiency. Perhaps the protein change provides a selective advantage. As a hypothetical example, maybe the mutated protein in question leads to a more efficient form of an intestinal binding protein specific for a trace nutrient that is important in sperm motility. This provides an easy visualization of how a beneficial trait will be selected for by nature.

Many people use the term *mutation*, but as I have said, not all mutations are deleterious, so the term *polymorphism* is more appropriate to use and simply means variant.

If you examine the genetic code within any population, you will find an enormous amount of variation. This stems from mutations and provides the fodder for the process of natural selection first described by Charles Darwin. Of course, although Darwin made his deductions from an examination of whole organisms, we are examining the same phenomenon, but from a molecular perspective. Maintaining population variation by natural selection alone is unlikely, because much of the variation within a population is selectively neutral, and subject to random change or what evolutionary biologists refer to as "drift." Drift is interesting because it can promote or eradicate extremely rare traits, particularly in small populations, which relates to the founder effect described earlier. In North America, the Anabaptist Amish and Hutterite communities give recent human examples of small culturally isolated populations that grew in size, and that now have a unique genetic signature with unrepresentative gene frequencies. The Amish grew from a founder population of around 200 and the Hutterites from 443 people. Both communities were closed to immigration. As a further example, Dutch immigrants arrived in South Africa during the seventeenth century, and although they were a small group, they were interesting in that they carried several rare genetic disorders that were not representative of the parent population from which they were drawn. The Dutch Afrikaner population grew rapidly and maintained the high frequency of these abnormal genetic traits. For example, a single couple of émigrés from Holland in the 1680s is now responsible for around 30,000 Afrikaners carrying the trait for porphyria variegata.

In the new synthesis of neo-Darwinian evolution, selection is examined in the context of how it acts on the fundamental genetic unit—the allele. We inherit a copy of any given gene from each of our parents. If neither copy (allele) contains, for example, an A where there is normally a G, then the genotype is wildtype. If one allele contains an A and the other allele a G, the genotype is referred to as heterozygous. If both alleles contain the abnormal (mutant) A, the genotype is homozygous recessive. By considering the frequency of polymorphic alleles, we can look at genetic evolution in a quantitative manner. For example, it is possible to work out how many generations it would take for a given level of selection pressure to substitute one allele for another. This is different to the view many people have of natural selection, because we are looking at the selection of molecular rather than phenotypic traits. As a consequence, scientists are now very interested in the relatively new idea of "selfish genes." Selfish genes and not phenotypes or genotypes span the generations. Consider that phenotypes senesce and die, whereas genotypes are determined as a function of meiosis—only the allele is immortal.

There is considerable debate as to the relative contribution of the following three phenomena as drivers of human evolution: (1) mutational induction of new alleles, (2) drift leading to selectively neutral random changes in allele frequency, and (3) natural selection forcing directional allele change. To put the importance of these evolutionary mechanisms into perspective, what makes us unique as individuals is the subtle, yet extensive variation in our genetic codes. There are in fact several alleles for any given gene in the human genome, emphasizing the seemingly infinite number of possibilities for individuality.

When wildtype and homozygous recessive genotypes are less fit than heterozygotes, then both wildtype and mutant alleles will be maintained in a population. This is known as a heterozygote advantage or balanced selection. The example that is always given to demonstrate this phenomenon describes how a valine substitution for glutamic acid in the hemoglobin molecule can protect individuals from sickle cell anemia. The "mutant" Hb$S$ allele is particularly common where malaria is endemic because heterozygosity (Hb$A$Hb$S$) for this trait protects against this life-threatening parasitic infection. Although wildtype (Hb$A$Hb$A$) individuals are less able to contend with *falcoparium* malaria, homozygous recessive individuals (Hb$S$Hb$S$) suffer from overt sickle cell anemia, a debilitating and often lethal condition. Despite this awful condition, the frequency of Hb$S$Hb$S$ individuals in parts of Africa within the malaria belt can reach 4% of the population. Clearly, the advantages of maintaining heterozygosity for this trait within the population are high. Another example of the heterozygote advantage is given by Tay–Sachs disease in which heterozygosity may confer a degree of protection against tuberculosis despite the recessive genotype being fatal by age 4. However, one of the most interesting and perhaps bizarre examples of a putative heterozygote advantage is given later in a discussion of human prion disease and cannibalism (see Chapter 7).

### 1.1.5   Population Genetics and the Hardy–Weinberg Equilibrium

If we want to examine allelic frequency within a population, and the forces that impact upon and change either the frequency of gene alleles or the genotypes, we can. The Hardy–Weinberg equilibrium permits us to calculate the expected genotype frequency from the allele frequency within the same population and the allele frequency from the known genotype. To accomplish this, we make certain assumptions: Mating occurs at random; reproductive efficiency is constant; no mutations are occurring; there is no effect on the population and its genotypes through selection pressure; and there is no effect on the population and its genotypes through inward or outward migration.

If we apply the Hardy–Weinberg equation, and the population we are studying does not fit Hardy–Weinberg predictions, then we have substantial evidence that some force like natural selection is acting on the population.

Hardy–Weinberg equation:

$$p^2 + 2pq + q^2 = 1$$

As a first step to see whether a population fits the Hardy–Weinberg equation, we need to calculate the allele frequencies. Let's look at this with some real data generated in the author's laboratory. 5,10-methylenetetrahydrofolate reductase (5,10MTHFR) is a folic acid-dependent enzyme that exists in polymorphic form. It is discussed extensively later in this book because it exhibits an important nutrient–gene interaction that impacts upon occlusive vascular disease, cancer, and birth defects. 5,10MTHFR helps regulate both DNA and homocysteine metabolism. The gene encoding 5,10MTHFR exhibits a common C-to-T substitution at nucleotide 677 (this is often written as 677C $\rightarrow$ T MTHFR or C677T-MTHFR). The C-to-T substitution at nucleotide 677 converts an alanine to a valine residue in the functional protein. This kind of polymorphism is often referred to as a single nucleotide polymorphism or SNP.

The possible genotypes are therefore wildtype—CC; heterozygote—CT; and homozygote recessive—TT. In a population of control patients recruited into a study to examine how this gene influenced vascular disease, we counted 41 CC, 46 CT, and 14 TT individuals. We can measure the allele frequency easily. Simply add the number of copies of each allele in the control population, and express it as a frequency. Remember that the population is diploid, and therefore, individuals have $2N$ alleles; the heterozygote has, as an example, one C allele and one T allele. Therefore, the frequency of the C allele is given by

$$(n_{CT} + 2n_{CC})/2N$$

Therefore, in our control population, $46 + 82/202 = 0.63$.

The frequency of the wildtype MTHFR-677C allele is 0.63, and by default, the frequency of the mutant MTHFR-677T allele is 0.37.

The frequency we obtain for the wildtype C allele is referred to as $p$, whereas the corresponding non-$p$ allele frequency is termed $q$. As I have shown above, $p + q = $ unity. We can use this information to work out the expected genotype frequencies as predicted by the Hardy–Weinberg equation. If we examine the two alleles C and T that have frequencies of $p$ and $q$, respectively, then we can expect a CC wildtype frequency of $p^2$, a CT heterozygote frequency of $2pq$, and a TT recessive homozygote frequency of $q^2$. Thus, $p^2 + 2pq + q^2 = 1(0.63^2 + 2(0.63 \times 0.37) + 0.37^2 = 1$.

This equation shows that when the frequency of a mutant allele is very low, the occurrence of the recessive homozygous genotype is extremely low, as in many rare genetic diseases. In the case of such rare genetic diseases, the mutant alleles tend to be concealed within heterozygotes where they are not expressed, so selection pressures cannot act against them. Consider this in the context of allele immortality as alluded to earlier.

As mentioned, nature acts to distort the idealized frequencies that are predicted by the Hardy–Weinberg equation. Some causes of this include:

- Ingress of migrants with a different allele frequency
- Natural selection against fertility or against survival to reproductive age of a certain genotype
- Subpopulation mating—in extreme situations, inbreeding
- Mutations creating new alleles
- Drift

The usual way to compare an observed genotype frequency with an expected one, assuming the Hardy–Weinberg equilibrium holds, is to perform a chi-square test for goodness of fit.

## 1.2 THE INHERITANCE OF GENETIC PACKETS OF INFORMATION

When alleles are juxtaposed on the DNA molecule, they are usually inherited together and do not segregate. The typical packet of genetic information that is inherited as a consequence of meiotic recombination might typically contain in excess of 20,000 base pairs.

Any given packet of genetic information will contain many polymorphisms. These SNPs are considered to be in linkage disequilibrium (LD). That is they are nonrandomly associated with nearby alleles. LD is associated with the physical distance on the DNA molecule between the loci of alleles, and it is under the variable influence of recombination.

A single packet of genetic information is referred to as a haplotype. Haplotype size within a population varies according to meiotic recombination, such that where ancestral human populations that are large in number, and have remained so for a significant period, will in all probability have smaller haplotypes (shorter DNA packets) and hence a lower LD. This stems from the greater number of genetic influences (mutations and recombinations) that have occurred in such populations and the effect that these events have on LD decay.

In the context of what follows on the ascent of man, African populations exhibit a larger number of haplotypes and more diverse LD patterns than non-African humans, who have evolved from small founder groups into new environments that differ significantly from the ancestral one. This greater genetic diversity among African populations is consistent with the view that modern man emerged out of an African evolutionary crucible.

Scientists also often refer to the "molecular clock" when investigating the evolutionary past and its various processes. To establish molecular dates, it is necessary to quantify the genetic distance between species, and then use a calibration rate such as the number of genetic changes expected per unit time. This permits one to convert genetic distance to time. Sophisticated models for achieving this include maximum likelihood (4,5) and Bayesian approaches (6). At the end of the day, the reliability of all molecular clock methods and their ability to provide information on the mechanisms that drive molecular evolution depends on the accuracy of the estimated genetic distance and the appropriateness of the calibration rate. See the panel on mitochondrial DNA (mtDNA) and elucidating "Eve."

## 1.3  A BRIEF OVERVIEW OF EVOLUTIONARY BIOLOGY AND THE ASCENT OF MAN

How can one briefly overview such a topic when it is possible to write volumes on the subject? In an excellent and fairly concise review of the "Genetics and making of *Homo sapiens*," which appeared in the journal *Nature* (7), the author, Sean Carroll, cites a passage from Shakespeare:

> What is man,
> If his chief good and the market of his time
> Be but to sleep and feed? A beast, no more.
> Sure, he that made us with such large discourse,
> Looking before and after, gave us not
> That capability and god-like reason
> To fust in us unused

> —W. Shakespeare, Hamlet IV:iv

We recognize that all human races presently on Earth are part of the same species, and that around 4 million years ago, a hominoid ape-like ancestor evolved out into three lineages—chimpanzees, gorillas, and early humans. Perhaps the best-known artifact from this time was discovered at Hadar, Ethiopia, and has been affectionately named "Lucy." Lucy is almost 4 million years old, and although she seems to be built in a robust ape-like manner, she was bipedal and walked upright on two legs as we do today.

It seems likely that bipedalism evolved early as a mechanism to free hands for the dexterous manipulation of tools and weaponry. Many of the attributes that man evolved such as increased intellect and brain size are discussed later in this book in the context of nutrition. Some of the oldest stone tools date back 2.5 million years and are associated with the fossils of our bipedal ancestor, *Homo habilis*. A million years later, the early human brain had enlarged and permitted the development of more highly refined tools.

These evolved characteristics are associated with *Homo erectus*. This species began a migration out of Africa about three quarters of a million years ago. However, within Africa, *Homo erectus* continued to evolve into modern man (*Homo sapiens*). This process was complete by around 100,000 to 200,000 years ago. *Homo sapiens* then migrated out from Africa and eventually supplanted *Homo erectus*. This simple view ignores the possibility that subspecies may have existed.

The cold climate that prevailed during the quaternary ice age in Eurasia probably gave rise to the Neanderthals (*Homo neanderthalensis*). These stoutly built people had heavy brow ridges above their eyes and were well evolved to survive the cold. They lived from 120,000 to 35,000 years ago and are considered to be *Homo sapiens*. Although they had extremely large brains, and well-evolved cultural practices, they eventually gave way to Cro-Magnon man who had appeared right across Europe by 35,000 years ago. This is a parallel time frame to the colonization of Asia and Australasia by what one would consider to be an anatomically modern form of *Homo sapiens* (Figures 1.4 and 1.5).

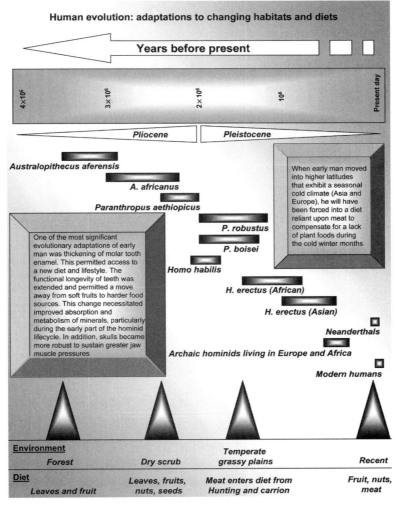

**Figure 1.4.** *The exposure of ancestral man to changing habitats and hence diets over the past 4 million years has played a role in our evolution as a species.*

**Mitochondrial DNA—The Search for Eve**

Human cells contain small organelles that are responsible for transducing sugar and oxygen into energy (ATP) with an unfortunate accumulation of reactive oxygen species as a toxic by-product of this respiratory process.

These organelles are known as mitochondria and contain a small amount of DNA (mtDNA). This DNA encodes 13 proteins required by the mitochondria as well as a large amount of non-coding DNA.

MtDNA provides an excellent molecular clock for very recent human history because of three characteristics:
1. Mitochondrial genes are only inherited maternally; that is, both males and females get their mitochondria from the female gamete.
2. Genetic recombination is not a general feature of mtDNA. This means that all contemporary populations alive today have an exact (barring novel mutations) copy of the mtDNA of a single woman living sometime in our past—a woman biologists refer to as "Eve."
3. mtDNA accrues mutations at a faster rate than nuclear DNA. It is because of this that mtDNA provides better resolution as a molecular clock than does nuclear chromosomal DNA and, hence, provides the best dating mechanism for our very recent history (the past few million years).

Careful examination of mtDNA in extant human populations allows us to estimate that all humankind may have descended from a single human female (Eve) that lived 200,000 years ago.

Controversy exists as to whether this date for Eve is correct, and if the detail regarding our African origins is true. Different models exist to explain our origins—these include replacement and multiregional models of human evolution.

**Figure 1.5.** *The concept of mitochondrial Eve is based on the molecular clock inherent in the maternal mitochondrial genome. The clock allows us to trace the female lineage back to the original ancestor of modern man.*

We will never know the complete story of our recent past, but there is consensus that as our brains grew, so to did our ability to produce and use tools and weapons. The skills to do this are necessarily learned. The ability to pass on and acquire such important information for survival probably acted as a driving force for the natural selection of intelligence, effective communication, and hence language. It is interesting to note, however, that the left–right asymmetry in Broca's area of the frontal lobe of the neo-cortex, an area that is associated with language ability, occurs in chimpanzees, bonobos, and gorillas, as well as in humans. This means the neuro-anatomical substrate of left-hemisphere dominance for speech was in place before the origin of hominins (7,8). Wernicke's posterior receptive language area in the temporal lobe is responsible for speech and gesture, as well as for musical talent, and again shows left-hemisphere dominance. Evidence from *Homo erectus* and *Homo neanderthalensis* endocasts as well as from chimpanzees show the presence of this shared asymmetry, again indicating its presence before the divergence of hominins.

From a physical viewpoint, the trend in the evolution of modern man was toward larger body mass, larger brains, longer legs relative to trunk, and smaller dentition. At a subtler, molecular level, the genetics of human evolution are of tremendous interest and yet, at the same time, are extraordinarily complex. With technological advances, however, we are now able to gain a far better idea of exactly what we are and how we came about (Figures 1.6–1.8).

## 1.4 THE –*OMICS* REVOLUTION

The new technologies that embrace the term –*omics* have evolved to address increasingly complex biological questions arising out of the postgenomics era. I describe some of these advanced techniques toward the end of this book. Briefly they encompass techniques like DNA microarray technology, real-time polymerase chain reaction, denaturing hplc, two-dimensional (2-D) protein electrophoresis coupled with matrix-assisted laser desorption/ionization–time-of-flight (MALDI–TOF) mass spectrometry, and *in silico* bioinformatics. These state-of-the-art techniques permit us to venture into the world of proteomics, transcriptomics, metabolomics, nutrigenomics, methylomics, and perhaps at the ultimate level to understand the "interactome." The interactome is defined as the sum of all protein interactions in the cell. A graphical representation of a typical "interaction map" looks like a massive aggregated collection of hairy dandelion seeds and is hugely complex (Figure 1.9). Such interactomes are often simplified into "functional interaction maps" in which proteins are allocated to functional categories (i.e., protein degradation, carbohydrate metabolism, and signal transduction). This provides a simpler three-dimensional (3-D) rendering of the network of cellular functions.

At the leading edge of scientific endeavor, it is becoming increasingly difficult to pigeonhole one's research interest. This book is a prime example of how interests in food, nutrition, genetics, molecular biology, clinical medicine, evolutionary theory, and anthropology come together to address the most fundamental of all human questions: "What does being human mean, and how did the condition arise?" Essentially, what is the meaning of life?

As an educator within our university system, I became frustrated by the notion that human nutrition is simply all about food, its constituents, and how they prevent disease or contribute, to it. As this book proves, nutrition is a far more diverse and philosophically deep subject than many students (and educators) think, and one that has never been more relevant than it is today. The two novel subdisciplines within nutrition that are now increasingly important are nutrigenomics and nutritional genetics. Peter Gillies (9) has defined these terms as follows: "Nutrigenomics refers to the prospective analysis of differences among nutrients with regard to the regulation of gene expression. In this context, nutrigenomics is a discovery science driven by the paradigms of molecular biology, enabled by microarray technology, and integrated on an informatics platform" (10,11). Gillies goes on to define nutrigenetics, or what many people refer to as nutritional genetics, as "the retrospective analysis of genetic variations among individuals with regard to their clinical response to specific nutrients. In this context, nutrigenetics is an applied science driven by the paradigms of

# The Rise of Modern Man:
## "Out of Africa Replacement" or a "Multiregional" Evolution?

### The Concepts:

The "Eve" hypothesis to support an "out of Africa" model for human evolution has much to commend it; this "out of Africa replacement" scenario is based on the molecular relatedness between African groups from within the continent, and between groups from Africa and other regions. The "out of Africa replacement model" assumes a human population originated in Africa 150,000 years ago with Eve as its source, and then radiated out, supplanting other human groups en route. However, this is only one possible option to account for our origins. An alternative model proposes that modern man evolved slowly from ancestral humans in many different areas of the world. This is the "multiregional model". This paradigm is based on populations gradually evolving into modern humans in many different locations. Implicit in this model is that differences in physiognomy (skin and hair color, build, etc.) between geographically distinct human populations have a longer adaptive chronology than would be implied by an "out of Africa" model. A third paradigm exists — "the assimilation model" contends that our origins were in fact African, but regional groups of archaic humans like the Neanderthals made a substantive contribution to our existing gene pool.

### The Evidence:

The debate between replacement (perhaps more logically referred to as uniregional) and multiregional models remains to be resolved: In a 2002 review, Satta and Takahata s1 weigh up the evidence for both models and conclude that the uniregional model is the most likely option to have occurred. Similarly, a recent 2005 paper by Ray and colleagues s2 describes the use of multilocus genetic data to infer the geographic origin of humans and distinguish between uni- and multiregional models. Using 377 genetic markers, they claim that East Africa is the most likely place of origin for modern humans and the source of human expansion into the Old World. However, Eswaran and colleagues s3 prefer a model in which the modern human phenotype originated in Africa and then advanced globally by local demic diffusion, hybridization, and natural selection. This phenotypic sweep represents an intermediate between the uniregional model (sweep of new species) and the multiregional model (independent single-locus selective sweeps). Overall, the emphasis of research findings, however, does seem to be toward a uniregional approach. Caramelli and coworkers S4 have typed ancient DNA sequences from Cro-Magnon man and found variability similar to contemporary humans, but at variance to the chronologically similar Neanderthals, indicating genetic discontinuity that makes it difficult to reconcile that both Neanderthals and early humans contributed to the current European gene pool. Some problems in evaluating the evidence are highlighted in a paper by Collard and Franchino S5. They suggest that the difficulties of pair-wise difference analysis of morphological/fossil data cannot be used to generate reliable estimates of primate phylogeny. Rather, molecular phylogeny is a more robust marker. Clearly, a consensus view on our origins is not easy to arrive at. It has been suggested that an exclusive focus on mtDNA has led to a one-sided and hence misleading picture of modern human origins that emphasizes a migration out of Africa with replacement s6. It is, however, difficult to ignore that, given limited variation within nonrecombined sequences of the autosomes, there is insufficient power to distinguish between models of human origin. Where autosomal loci do exhibit the required resolution, they point to the uniregional model S7. One thing is sure, though, this important debate on our origins is likely to continue into the foreseeable future.

**Specific references to this subject:**
S1 Satta Y. & Takahata N. Out of Africa with regional interbreeding? Modern human origins. Bioessays 2002; 24: 871-5.
S2 Ray N, Currat M, Berthier P, & Excoffier L. Recovering the geographic origin of early modern humans by realistic and spatially explicit simulations. Genome Res 2005; 15: 1161-7.
S3 Eswaran V. & Harpending H. Rogers AR. Genomics refutes an exclusively African origin of humans. J Hum Evol 2005; 49: 1-18.
S4 Caramelli D, Lalueza-Fox C, Vernesi C, et al. Evidence for a genetic discontinuity between Neanderthals and 24,000-year-old anatomically modern Europeans. Proc Natl Acad Sci U S A 2003;100: 6593-7. Epub 2003 May 12.
S5 Collard M. & Franchino N. Pairwise difference analysis in modern human origins research. J Hum Evol 2002; 43: 323-52.
S6 Harpending H. & Eswaran V. Tracing modern human origins. Science 2005; 309: 1995.
S7 Macaulay V, Hill C, Achilli A, et al. Tracing modern human origins. Science 2005; 309: 1995.

*Figure 1.6.* Contemporary theories to explain the recent ascent of humankind are based on two models: an "out of Africa replacement model" in which we evolved as a species in Africa, and radiated out to colonize the planet, and a model in which "multiregional evolution" of our species occurred.

# Out of Africa pattern of human migration—The African replacement hypothesis

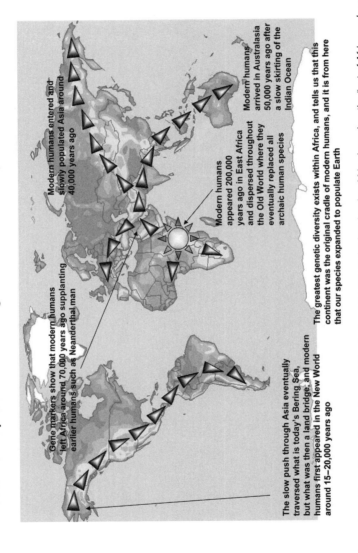

**Figure 1.7.** *This figure shows the pattern of migratory radiation that our species took when leaving Africa based on the "out of Africa replacement model," which is the favored paradigm for our recent evolutionary past.*

## A small and very old lady from Flores provides human evolutionary biologists with a dilemma

In late 2004, the unearthing of an 18,000-year-old skeleton at Liang Bua on the Eastern Indonesian island of Flores has presented a significant paradox for evolutionary biologists to ponder [S1, S2]. The discovery of tiny, 1-m-tall hominins, nicknamed "hobbits" by their discoverers, but more correctly termed *Homo floriensis* brought to the worlds attention a species with a brain roughly one third the size of that of modern man's. However, despite such a small brain, it seems that this new species of hominin had very large temporal lobes, a character normally associated with auditory and speech recognition. Furthermore, *Homo floriensis* had substantial convolutions of the frontal lobes indicating an ability for higher cognition. So, despite a small brain, these diminutive hominins may have been capable of shaping and using stone tools, a characteristic normally reserved for prehistoric modern man, rather than earlier hominins [S3].

The important finding here is that *Homo floriensis* may defy our long-held beliefs relating to the evolution of the human brain. Specifically, advanced behavioral traits and the creation and use of stone implements do not require an anatomically modern brain—the same outcome may be achieved simply by rewiring and increasing the convolutions of a smaller brain. Little comparability was found between endocasts derived from *Homo floriensis* and those of the modern human pygmy and abnormal microcephalic brains, and so the anatomical structure of the *Homo floriensis* brain challenges accepted wisdom on the importance of brain size.

The second interesting deduction is that the tiny stature of *Homo floriensis* suggests humans are as readily influenced by evolutionary forces as are any other species: The genetic isolation of *Homo floriensis* on Flores led to selection pressures shrinking this hominin to dwarf proportions due to the limited resources on this Indonesian island. Clearly, as a genus, *Homo* is far more adaptive in terms of its morphological response to ecological determinants, such as food availability, than we had previously thought possible.

The recent discovery of *Homo floriensis* along with many other new taxa raises a third point: The origin, number, antiquity, and morphological characteristics of several recent discoveries relating to the fossil hominin record have led to a call for an alternative viewpoint on paleoanthropology's fundamental "out of Africa" paradigm S4. It certainly seems that our recent evolution is neither clear cut nor is it fully understood.

*Specific references to this subject:*
S1. Brown P, Sutikna T, Morwood MJ, et al. A new small-bodied hominin from the Late Pleistocene of Flores, Indonesia. Nature 2004; 431: 1043–4
S2. Morwood MJ, Soejono RP, Roberts RG, et al Archaeology and age of a new hominin from Flores in eastern Indonesia. Nature 2004; 431: 1087–91
S3. Balter M. Paleoanthropology. Small but smart? Flores hominid shows signs of advanced brain. Science 2005; 307: 1386-9.
S4. Dennell R. & Roebroeks W. An Asian perspective on early human dispersal from Africa. Nature 2005; 438: 1069-104.

**Figure 1.8.** *The 2004 discovery of* Homo floriensis *on the Indonesian island of Flores challenges our perceived wisdom relating to man's recent evolutionary past.*

## A simple representation of an interactome

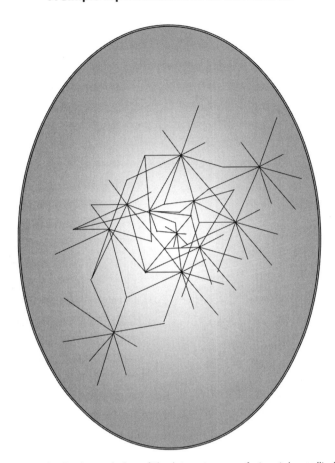

**Figure 1.9.** *An extremely simple rendering of the interactome; unfortunately, reality is infinitely more complex than can be represented here. Imagine each node as a cluster of proteins with similar cellular function. Each cluster is then linked by an interactive network. As an example, three juxtaposed nodes in the above figure might represent DNA synthesis proteins, DNA repair proteins, and cell-cycle regulatory proteins. Then consider a hypothetical node for proteins involved in protein folding; these are likely to be located at a more distant nexus as they are not closely involved with the former three protein clusters. Now imagine how complex an interactome for humans would be if each protein represented a single node!*

nutritional pharmacology in the context of genetic polymorphisms and clinical experience." These are sound definitions, and worthy of reiteration for all students of the subject.

As our knowledge of the "nutriome" improves and the gaps within the interactome are filled in, it seems likely that the buzzwords of today like nutrigenomics and nutritional genetics will ultimately give way to the unifying field of human molecular nutrition.

# Chapter 2

# *Molecular Mechanisms of Genetic Variation Linked to Diet*

## 2.1 A BRIEF HISTORY OF THE HUMAN DIET

Early man met his needs for macro- and micronutrients via a largely herbivorous diet (12). It has been postulated that as man moved toward a more nutrient-dense diet, this facilitated an increase in brain dimension with a concomitant decrease in gut size (13). Such a diet was likely to contain not just animal fat and protein but plants (leaves/shoots/roots/berries). Clearly, a significant mismatch exists between our ancestral diet and our contemporary one, which is energy rich-nutrient poor. This book examines not just some of the more interesting nutritional selection pressures that forged our species, and that are dealt with in this chapter, but it will also attempt to examine how incompatibility between programming in our ancestral genes and the dietary consequences of an agricultural revolution has led to the evolution of chronic debilitating human diseases within modern society (Figure 2.1).

## 2.2 THE ROLE OF MILK IN HUMAN EVOLUTION

It has been suggested that lactation evolved as the most advantageous way to provide infant nutrition when food was unavailable or patchy, despite inefficiencies associated with converting nutrients from food to reserves and milk (14). One of the best nutrient-related examples of human genetic variation maintained via natural selection is given by our ability to digest milk lactose. Like most mammals, humans slowly lose their ability to digest lactose after weaning and have a low digestive capacity, which leads to abdominal discomfort when

*Molecular Nutrition and Genomics: Nutrition and the Ascent of Humankind*, by Mark Lucock
Copyright © 2007 John Wiley & Sons, Inc.

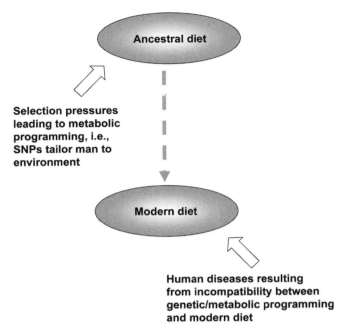

**Figure 2.1.** Incompatibility between programming in our ancestral genes and the dietary consequences of a modern diet.

in excess of 500 mL of milk is consumed. By contrast, many northern Europeans, northern Africans, and Arab populations maintain their ability to digest lactose into adulthood, and they have a high digestive capacity. The dominant *LAC P* gene controls adult lactose digestion: Either one or two alleles confer high digestive capacity. By contrast, homozygosity for the recessive allele *LAC R* confers low digestive capacity. The genetic distribution of *LAC P* may stem from the environmental pressures of a nomadic lifestyle in some northern African and Arab populations.

Nomads from this part of the world probably came to rely on goat and camel milk during the drier months; to obtain all their fluid, energy, and protein requirements, they would need to exceed the threshold 500-mL value by a factor of at least 5×. This large volume of milk would have to be consumed while fresh, and as a consequence, the *LAC P* allele has a high frequency in today's nomadic tribes from this region. Quite simply, this gene probably facilitated survival. The Beja of the desert region between the Nile and the Red Sea exhibit milk dependence sufficient to result in selective pressures in favor of the lactase persistence allele. The proportion of lactose malabsorbers was 16.8% in the Beja and 74.5% in the Nilotes of Sudan who are semi-nomadic cattle herders. The high prevalence of lactose malabsorption among the Nilotes fits into a converging gradient of lactase gene frequencies along the Nile Valley (15). Rationalizing this simple nutrient–gene interaction that permits survival in an extreme environment is straightforward, but why is the lactase persistence allele common in the United Kingdom and other northern European countries? It has been suggested that substantial geographic coincidence exists among (1) high diversity in dairy cattle genes, (2) locations of the European Neolithic cattle farming sites (>5000 years ago), and (3) present-day lactose tolerance in Europeans. This suggests a gene-culture coevolution between cattle and humans (16).

Another hypothesis suggests that having an ability to digest lactose increases vitamin D absorption. At northern European latitudes, the level of ultraviolet (UV) exposure is insufficient to manufacture vitamin D all year round. Lactose tolerance may therefore help prevent the vitamin D deficiency disease rickets as well as maintain key biochemical interactions involving vitamin D within the cell nucleus (see below).

It is interesting to note the irony that, after returning from his voyage in the Beagle in 1836, Charles Darwin suffered from long bouts of abdominal discomfort that perplexed his physicians for 40 years. Darwin only recovered, when, by chance, he refrained from milk and cream. Darwin's malady highlights the importance of lactose in mammalian and human evolution in a somewhat obtuse, but nonetheless salient, manner (17).

## 2.3 MICRONUTRIENTS AND THE EVOLUTION OF SKIN PIGMENTATION

Two key micronutrients may have played a critical role in the evolution of skin coloration. Pigmentation with melanin is an adaptive response that is maintained by natural selection. The vitamin D hypothesis states that pale skins were necessary outside tropical latitudes to facilitate vitamin D biosynthesis within the skin from low levels of UV light. Thus, depigmentation evolved as humankind radiated out of the tropics where a dark skin protected against excess, even toxic, synthesis of vitamin D (18). More recently, Jablonski and Chaplin (19) formulated a superbly elegant paradigm to show how degradation of UV labile folic acid (20) might impair reproductive success by destroying a molecule critical to cell division (Figures 2.2 and 2.3), and that arresting vitamin $D_3$ synthesis in the skin at high latitudes could further impair reproductive success by altering calcium homeostasis (Figure 2.4). They conclude that natural selection has produced two opposing clines of skin coloration. One based on folate that *photoprotects* in a gradation from dark pigmentation at the equator to fair skin at the poles. The second cline, based on vitamin $D_3$ *photosynthesis*, shows a gradation from low pigmentation at the poles to dark coloration at the equator. At the central nexus of these two clines, populations exhibit an increased capability for developing facultative pigmentation to cope with changing seasonal UV levels.

Of course, skin pigmentation is multifactorial with genes such as MC1R (melanocortin-1 receptor gene), in particular, being a major determinant of skin and hair pigmentation (21). This gene is highly polymorphic in fair-skinned populations, but less so in dark-skinned African populations (19). Other genes such as MATP (membrane-associated transporter protein) contain SNPs that are also strongly associated with variation in human pigmentation (22). However, it is also worthy to note that wholly intracellular folates in the form of tetrahydro-, 5,10-methylenetetrahydro-, or 10-formyltetrahydrofolate tend to be particularly labile, and these are the forms required for nucleotide biosynthesis and cellular replication (23). UV scission of these coenzymes may be particularly harmful in respect to reproductive efficiency. We have previously shown that UV-B light at 312 nm with a calculated energy of 91.78 kcal/mol profoundly enhances oxidation of monoglutamyl 5-methyltetrahydrofolate (plasma form of folate) to 5-methyldihydrofolate, with a subsequent and irreversible loss of vitamin activity via C9–N10 bond scission, forming a pterin residue and p-aminobenzoylglutamate (20). Recent research from the author's

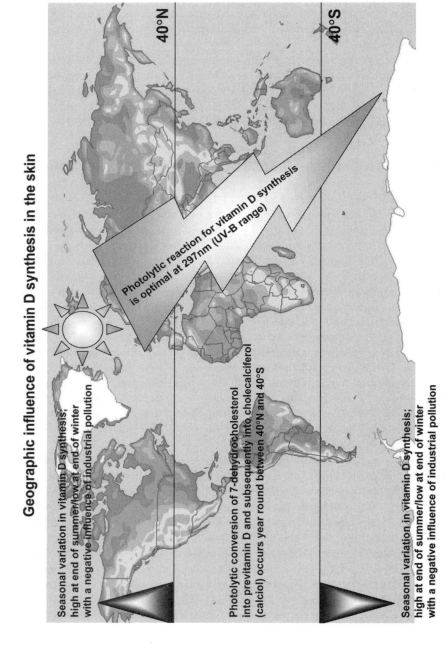

**Figure 2.2.** *Vitamin D is synthesized in our skin as a consequence of exposure to a specific wavelength of UV light (290–312 nm). As UV exposure varies with latitude, only people within 40° N and S of the equator synthesize this critical vitamin year round. Outside of these latitudes, vitamin D synthesis is seasonal. It has been suggested that this may have acted as an evolutionary pressure for skin depigmentation.*

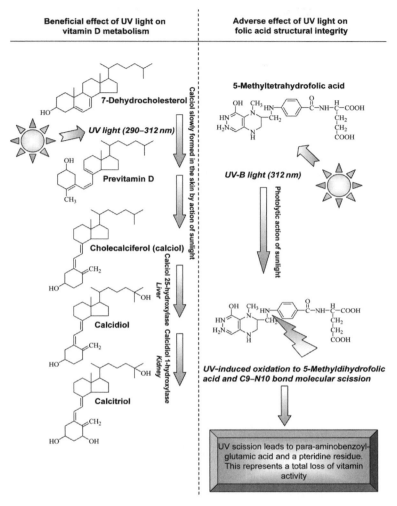

**Figure 2.3.** *It has been suggested that global variation in exposure to UV light may have acted as a selection pressure for skin pigmentation. Protection against the photolytic effect on labile folate, a molecule required for cell growth, division, and reproduction may have favored enhanced pigmentation as one moves toward the equator, whereas the reverse may be true for the necessary action of UV light on vitamin D synthesis, which could have led to depigmentation as one travels toward the poles. The figure shows the contrasting effect of UV light on the molecular structures of both folate and vitamin D.*

laboratory shows C9–N10 bond scission of the intracellular polyglutamyl form of 5-methyltetrahydrofolate may be even more pronounced. Furthermore, another vitamin—ascorbic acid (vitamin C)—is crucial for optimizing native folate bioavailabilty (Figure 2.5) (24), whereas dietary riboflavin (vitamin B$_2$) and cobalamin (vitamin B$_{12}$) are also crucial to the one-carbon transfer reactions that folate facilitates in its role of *de novo* methionine, purine, and pyrimidine synthesis (25). Indeed, the most important of all folate's covitamins, vitamin B$_{12}$, is highly UV sensitive, as is riboflavin. Clearly, many factors affect folate status and, hence, are likely to indirectly modulate the skin pigmentation evolutionary paradigm.

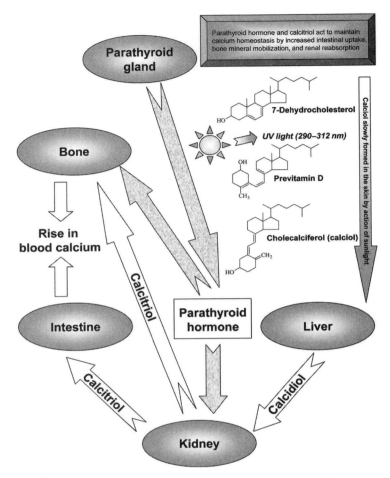

**Figure 2.4.** *A simple schematic of vitamin D and calcium homeostasis.*

A more indirect effect may lie in the role of closely related biopterin cofactors and melanin biosynthesis. Folate and biopterin coenzymes are structurally and functionally similar (Figure 2.6). Metabolic overlap is thought to occur between their respective pathways; man cannot synthesize folate *de novo*, but bacteria can. GTP cyclohydrolase 1 is used by bacteria for folate production, but it is also used by man for tetrahydrobiopterin biosynthesis (26). A common metabolic locus in both pathways, which is distinct in evolutionary terms, indicates a close metabolic relationship exists between both groups of cofactors and their dependent enzymes. Indeed, a reciprocal use of substrates has been reported. Melanin is formed from tyrosine; the first step is the formation of DOPA from tyrosine, a process that requires tetrahydrobiopterin (see below—Figure 4.1). Interestingly, folate and biopterin are known to interact in a synergistic manner at such sites (20,27–30), and they both may therefore play a role in melanogenesis, although this is unproven.

Nonmammalian vertebrate pigmentation may also advertise a capacity to deploy resources in a way that optimizes survival and reproductive success. Carotenoid precursors of vitamin A are used by birds to provide sexual coloration that advertises superior health as

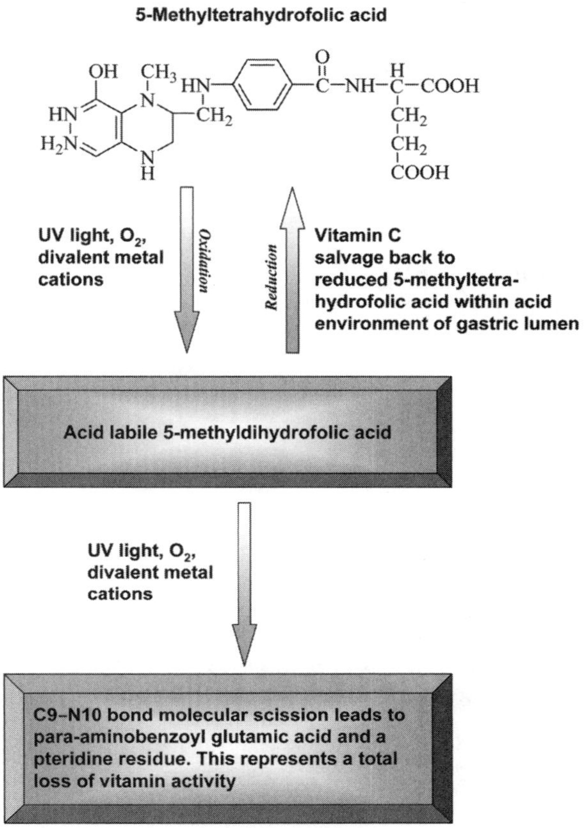

5-Methyltetrahydrofolic acid

**Figure 2.5.** Schematic showing that vitamin C is crucial for optimizing native folate bioavailabilty.

conferred by the antioxidant properties of carotenoids (31). However, several micronutrients with specific epigenetic and antioxidant capacity also undoubtedly help maintain genetic integrity and thus reproductive success in humans (see below).

## 2.4 MICRONUTRIENTS OPTIMIZE GAMETOGENESIS AND REPRODUCTIVE FECUNDITY

Important epigenetic phenomena associated with folate status and metabolism, coupled with the observed increase in sperm counts after selenium, zinc, and folate supplementation in both fertile and infertile men have led to the suggestion that adequate nutritional intake of folate, selenium, and zinc may be important for male fecundity (32–34). In common with well-recognized folate-linked developmental processes in pregnancy, the benefit of adequate folate nutrition in men is likely to be due to the improved robustness of nucleotide biosynthesis necessary to support all cellular processes dependent on the fidelity of DNA replication. The most likely effect of aberrant folate metabolism in spermatogenesis is the abnormal accumulation of damaged spermatozoal DNA (see below for mechanistic explanation of this general principle).

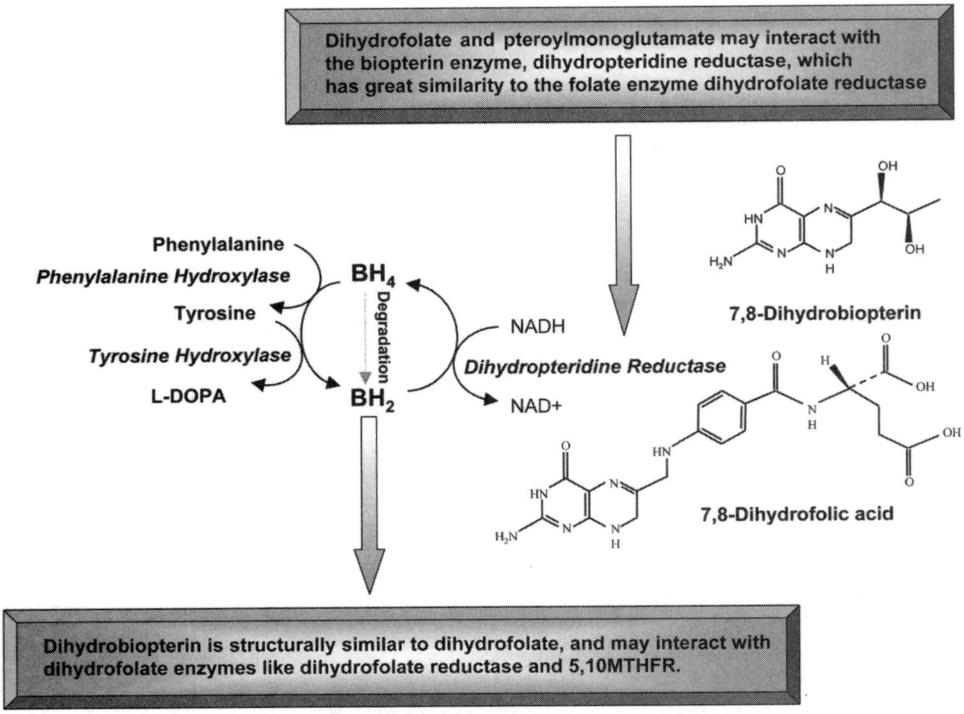

**Figure 2.6.** *Importance of biopterin in aromatic amino acid hydroxylase reactions, and putative ways in which folate and biopterin pathways may interact.*

## 2.4.1  Mechanisms of Selenium as an Evolutionary Pressure on Gametogenesis

Selenium is critically important in spermatogenesis, and it is incorporated in the sperm mitochondria capsule and may thus affect the behavior and function of the spermatozoon. In humans, information is contradictory; both low and high sperm selenium concentrations are reported to have a negative influence on the number and motility of spermatozoa (33). Selenium sits in the catalytic cleft of glutathione peroxidase in the form of selenocysteine, where it neutralizes free radicals. It is well recognized that selenium protects developing sperm from susceptibility to peroxidative damage as a consequence of spermatozoa's high polyunsaturated fatty acid level, inability to repair membrane damage, and high potential to generate DNA-damaging superoxide and hydrogen peroxide (34). Selenium deficiency in females may also be important, and it has been reported to result in infertility, abortions, and retention of the placenta (35).

Although selenium toxicity occurs at only moderate levels of this micronutrient, deficiency is widespread across parts of China, the United States, and Scandinavia. This means that the unique chemistry of selenocysteine residues in countering environmental stress may play a significant role in reproductive vigor, both in our recent history and in the present day. Indeed, UGA, the codon for selenocysteine, is the most interesting code word in the evolution of life as it has served more functions than any other codon (36). Figure 2.7 shows how selenium acts as an antioxidant at the level of glutathione peroxidase. However, clearly

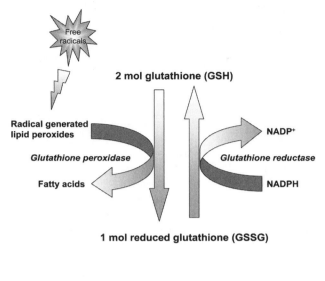

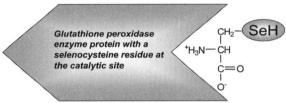

**Figure 2.7.** *Antioxidant role of selenium with reference to its function in maintaining glutathione peroxidase activity.*

many micronutrients and antioxidants also act to protect DNA from damage (see below) One of these, vitamin E, actually has a synergy with selenium in that vitamin E removes the products of lipid peroxidation, whereas selenium in the form of glutathione peroxidase reduces hydrogen peroxide to water and acts to remove the cause of lipid peroxidation, as well as to recycle the tocopheroxyl radical back into vitamin E ($\alpha$-tocopherol).

### 2.4.2 Mechanisms of Folate as an Evolutionary Pressure on Gametogenesis

In the context of nutrigenomics and gametogenesis, 5,10-methylenetetrahydrofolate and its dependent polymorphic enzyme 5,10-methylenetetrahydrofolate reductase (5,10MTHFR) are crucial intermediates in folate metabolism: Although 5,10-methylenetetrahydrofolate is used by the reductase to produce 5-methyltetrahydrofolate and *de novo* methionine (Figure 2.8), it is also required by both thymidylate synthase and methylenetetrahydrofolate dehydrogenase in the synthesis of DNA-thymine and purine, respectively. Thus, 5,10-methylenetetrahydrofolate is at the branch point for three important pathways (38), and its regulation by folate status and common variants of genes coding for folate dependent enzymes is clearly an important step in mammalian one-carbon metabolism. The 5,10MTHFR gene exhibits several SNPs, of which the common C677T-MTHFR variant is associated with higher risk for spina-bifida, Down's syndrome, and complications of pregnancy such as pre-eclampsia, recurrent early pregnancy loss, and fetal growth restriction. It is also an important factor in vascular disease. However, this SNP can also predispose or offer protection against certain conditions such as colon cancer, depending on nutritional status.

The probable explanation for this duality of effect is that the C677T-MTHFR polymorphism increases levels of 5,10-methylenetetrahydrofolate critical for nucleotide biosynthesis. Hence, with adequate folate nutrition, an accumulation of 5,10-methylenetetrahydrofolate might actually protect against developmental and embryological complications as well as many degenerative diseases. However, with poor folate nutrition, this same SNP might compromise cellular levels of 5,10-methylenetetrahydrofolate required for conversion of dUMP into dTMP and thus augment misincorporation of uracil into DNA, a process leading to genomic instability (39). Recent related research has shown that the DNA mismatch repair system responsible for maintaining genomic integrity and the apoptotic response (programmed cell death) is also sensitive to folate deficiency (40).

Given such profound mechanistic effects, it is perhaps not surprising that evidence suggests a survival advantage exists for fetuses homozygous for the C677T-MTHFR polymorphism, particularly where maternal folate levels are replete: It has been shown that a four-fold higher incidence of this SNP occurs in neonates compared with aborted fetuses (41). In support of this, the widespread implementation of periconceptional folate supplements over the last 20 years has led to an increase in the incidence of homozygous C677T-MTHFR individuals (42).

Considerably less is known about the role of folate–gene interactions with respect to the elaboration and epigenetic regulation of DNA in spermatogenesis and male fertility. We know that folate and zinc supplementation demonstrably improves sperm counts and sperm morphology in both fertile and infertile men (32), and that folate coenzymes stabilize C677T-MTHFR by preventing the polymorphic enzyme from relinquishing its flavin cofactor (43). Furthermore, as can be seen below and in Figure 2.8, and later in Figure 6.3, folate-derived methyl groups are additionally required for methylation of DNA-CpG groups that regulate gene expression. These facts, and the central role of folate in the elaboration of DNA, renders dietary folate a nutrient that may exert a significant selection pressure on human evolution during the periconceptional period (25) (see also *Direct Dietary Selection of a Human Metabolomic Profile*).

### 2.4.3 Iron as a Recent Evolutionary Pressure on Reproductive Fecundity

Early European populations are likely to have suffered from iron deficiency and consequently an increase in premature delivery and hence low birth-weight offspring (44,45). It has been demonstrated that hemochromatosis, a genetic disease associated with progressive iron overload, is associated with a C282Y mutation in the HLA-H gene. This gene has reached a high frequency in a short time (it arose around 60 generations ago (46,47)). This positive selection may well have improved the reproductive fitness of C282Y heterozygote carriers; 32% of females of reproductive age who were normal homozygotes for a hemochromatosis mutation had iron deficiency compared with only 21% of heterozygote females of reproductive age. A similar trend in iron deficiency exists for males (45). The deleterious effects of this condition are of late-onset (in the fifth or sixth decade of life), so it seems that C282Y, which represents 85% of all hemochromatosis mutations, may exert a selective advantage during the reproductive phase of the human lifecycle by lowering the complications of premature birth associated with low iron status.

Iron may play another important role in achieving a normal term pregnancy. Hypoxia inducible factor $1\alpha$ (HIF-$1\alpha$) is a component of the master transcription regulator (HIF) for genes that respond to hypoxia or iron deficiency. In the presence of oxygen and iron, proline residues in two degradation domains are altered by HIF-1-prolyl hydroxylases leading to ubiquitination and degradation of HIF-$1\alpha$. HIF-$1\alpha$ is thus stable in conditions lacking oxygen or iron (49). Pre-eclampsia (pregnancy induced hypertension) is the leading cause of fetal and maternal mortality worldwide. Vascular endothelial growth factor (VEGF) may be compromised in pre-eclamptic mothers. The pre-eclamptic placenta produces elevated levels of a soluble tyrosine kinase 1 receptor that catches free VEGF. This capture of VEGF compromises the vasculature of the kidney, brain lungs and other organs which are deprived of essential survival and maintenance signals, and hence dysfunction. This has been shown to lead on to hypertension and kidney disease in rodents, which mirrors human pre-eclampsia. Mice that lack one VEGF allele also develop the same pathology shown by pregnant women with pre-eclampsia (50). It is now thought that HIF-$1\alpha$ may have a protective role in regulating VEGF in pre-eclampsia. Degradation of HIF-$1\alpha$ during normoxia involves binding to von Hippel–Lindau (VHL) protein via the oxygen/iron-sensitive degradation domain mentioned above. It has been suggested that homozygosity for a C598T-VHL polymorphism originated from a single founder no more than 62,000 years ago, and it may have a survival advantage. Such an advantage may involve improvements in iron metabolism, erythropoiesis, embryonic development, energy metabolism, or modulation of risk for pre-eclampsia (51).

### 2.4.4  Phytoestrogens and Reproduction

Whether phytoestrogens found in many plant foods have played any role in reproductive success at a level that may have evolutionary implications is unclear. However, these isoflavones compete with endogenous estrogens such as estradiol for occupancy of the estrogen receptor (ER), which is common to many reproductive tissues. The bound ligand is responsible for activation of the genomic estrogen response element within the nucleus and, hence, protein expression. An excessive stimulation of ERs in reproductive tissue is associated with poor fecundity. This area is covered in more depth later.

## 2.5  DIRECT DIETARY SELECTION OF A HUMAN METABOLOMIC PROFILE

Some SNPs may have arisen in extant human populations to help deal with a particular dietary element in the most efficient and effective manner available. It seems highly likely that a global mosaic of ancestral dietary patterns may have acted as selection pressures that favored particular alleles or combinations of alleles in a way that could help steer metabolic processes to aid survival. The following discussion provides some examples.

### 2.5.1  Advantage of the Alanine: Glyoxylate Aminotransferase (AGT) Pro11Leu Polymorphism in Meat Eaters

AGT is an important enzyme in intermediary metabolism. A C-to-T substitution in the AGT gene leads to the Pro11Leu polymorphism, which causes a three-fold decrease in enzyme activity along with a small amount of protein mistargeted between organelles. The effect of this on the synthesis and excretion of oxalate and deposition of calcium oxalate crystals in the kidney and urinary tract is thought to be significant. It has been postulated that there is a distinct advantage to possession of this SNP for populations that are predominantly meat eaters. It is believed that redirection of a small proportion (ca. 5%) of AGT from peroxisomes to mitochondria in humans might lead to a subcellular partitioning of AGT that was better suited to an omnivorous as opposed to a herbivorous lifestyle (52) and, hence, offer meat eaters a distinct survival advantage. Caldwell et al. (53) recently showed that the frequency of Pro11Leu allelic frequency varied widely among 11 extant human populations with differing ancestral diets. The frequency varied from 27.9% in the Saami with a meat-rich ancestral diet to 2.3% in Chinese who have a more mixed ancestral diet. Using the genetic distance measure $F_{ST}$, these authors conclude that the frequency of this allele has been shaped by dietary selection pressure.

### 2.5.2   Contemporary Selection Pressure from Periconceptional Folate Supplements

Despite the enormous well-proven benefits of folate nutrition (54), recent findings suggest that exposure to elevated levels of this vitamin during the periconceptional period could select human embryos that carry the mutant 677T-MTHFR allele (20,25,55) (also see Figure 2.8 for explanation and further reference). It is recognized that in the presence of a low folate status, this mutant allele is associated with elevated homocysteine, and aberrant epigenetic processes, both of which are thought to be key factors in vascular disease and cancer (20,25). Additionally, when cellular levels of folate are low, this same SNP might compromise the accumulation of 5,10-methylenetetrahydrofolate and hence impair the conversion of dUMP into dTMP (Figures 2.8 and 2.9), and thus facilitate uracil misincorporation (56), leading to genomic instability. This provides a putative, yet elegant, explanation to account for the loss of the developing embryo. An accumulation of homocysteine may also compound this negative *in utero* effect (57); indeed, it has been proposed that homocysteine embryotoxicity results from an inhibition of transmethylation reactions, a consequence of increased embryonic s-adenosylhomocysteine levels (58). This may impact on CpG methylation patterns that regulate gene expression at a critical time point in embryonic development. However, with a folate status that is replete, an accumulation of 5,10-methylenetetrahydrofolate might actually protect against the misincorporation of uracil into DNA, and problems in the elaboration and subsequent stability of chromosomes. Taken collectively, the demographic and genetic information currently available on the 677T-MTHFR allele suggests a scenario whereby the TT genotype could actually increase an early embryo's viability where or when folate nutrition is adequate (20,25,55) (also see Figure 2.8 for explanation and further reference). This includes regions with an abundant supply of fresh green vegetables, and populations subject to folate supplements as a preventative measure against neural tube defect (i.e., spina bifida) affected pregnancy (25).

### 2.5.3   The Cost–Benefit Analysis of Polymorphisms within Lipoprotein Metabolism

Apolipoprotein E is central to blood lipoprotein homeostasis and lipid transport within tissues. The gene (APO-E) encoding this protein is polymorphic. Although the APO-E4 allele is a well-established risk factor for both vascular disease and Alzheimer's disease in

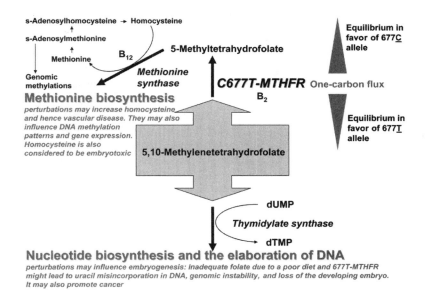

**Figure 2.8.** *Schematic showing the MTHFR locus, which is encoded by a variant C677T-MTHFR gene. The implication of the genetic selection of the MTHFR genotype, folate metabolism, and reproductive efficiency is dealt with in an important paper by Reyes-Engel et al. (37).*

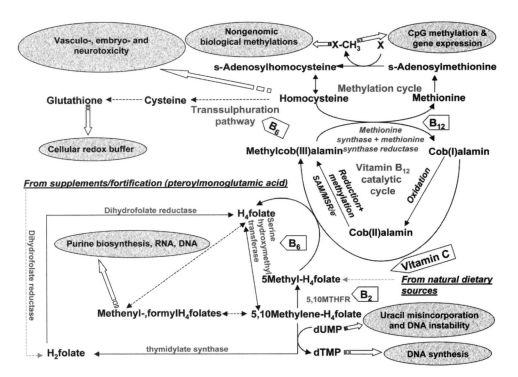

**Figure 2.9.** *Highly simplified schematic of folate-dependent processes. Includes locus of involvement for other vitamins.*

post-reproductive years, it may, however, in certain cultures/feeding modes, offer a distinct survival advantage. The common APO-E3 allele is found in all human populations, but it is particularly prevalent in long-established agricultural economies, such as persist around the Mediterranean Sea. This contrasts with the prevalence of the APO-E4 allele, which is highest in cultures that still have an economy based on foraging, or where food supply is unpredictable and scarce. Such populations include Pygmies, African Khoi San, Malaysian and Australian Aborigines, Papuans, Lapps, and Native Americans (59). Based on this distribution, it has been suggested that the ancestral APO-E4 allele may be a "thrifty" allele with functional properties that influence lipoprotein metabolism, including cholesterol levels in a beneficial manner in the appropriate ancestral environment. However, out of their ancestral context (i.e., within a contemporary environment where Western diets and longevity prevail) chronic degenerative diseases more readily manifest themselves (59). Although feeding mode may well have influenced metabolome selection in these populations, the APO-E polymorphism may also influence reproductive efficiency/fertility via the effect it has on cholesterol and hence steroidogenesis (60).

APO-E4 is not the only thrifty allele to influence cholesterol levels. Ancestral diets rich in fiber, vegetable protein, plant sterols, etc., were clearly low in *trans*-fatty acids and the other substrates of cholesterol biosynthesis (Figure 2.10). It has been suggested that, as a result, a range of cholesterol raising polymorphisms exist that have been conserved by evolution (61). These include the B2B2 genotype of the cholesteryl ester transfer protein-Taq1B, which favors cholesterol transfer to the liver for bile acid synthesis (62), and the T54 GA/AA genotypes of the intestinal fatty acid binding protein gene which favors fatty acid absorption for cholesterol synthesis (63). Clearly, a partial return to our ancestral diet of vegetables, fruit, and nuts would be an effective measure to reduce aberrant blood lipid profiles. Figure 2.10 shows how plant sterols like $\beta$-sitosterol are structurally similar to cholesterol and hence may competitively reduce cholesterol absorption.

### 2.5.4 "Thirsty" Genes—Putative Thrifty Genes that May Have Been Selected to Counter Water Stress, but Now Lead to Hypertension

Humans have a physiological requirement for salt and mineral sodium. Indeed, one of our most basic senses of taste is for saltiness. This taste is not unpleasant, and it is perhaps unsurprising that in the West, our salt intake far exceeds our physiologic needs. Even the U.S. Food and Drug Administration recommendation of 6 g/day for a low-salt diet is estimated to be 3.5× that of the typical Paleolithic diet. Some people are sensitive to salt and possess a genetic predisposition toward developing life-threatening hypertension (high blood pressure). Ten percent of people are affected by salt sensitivity in this way.

It has been suggested that our early hunter-gatherer ancestors survived on little salt. However, the agricultural revolution and urbanization led to an increase in salt usage with genetically predisposed individuals developing age-related hypertension (64). Lev-Ran and Porta (64) hypothesize that selection pressures may have favored the emergence of a salt-sensitive, hypertensive genotype. This they argue might have been a thrifty gene phenomenon, like the APO-E4 allele mentioned earlier, which supported energy savers in times of scarcity, but in contemporary society contributes to chronic degenerative disease. They suggest that "thirsty" genes may act on salt and water retention and, hence, helped early man survive the challenge of water volume depleting illnesses. This may have been useful under water stress situations, but it is deleterious in respect of causing hypertension in post-reproductive individuals in our aging contemporary societies.

**Structural similarity between plant sterols (β-sitosterol)
and cholesterol**

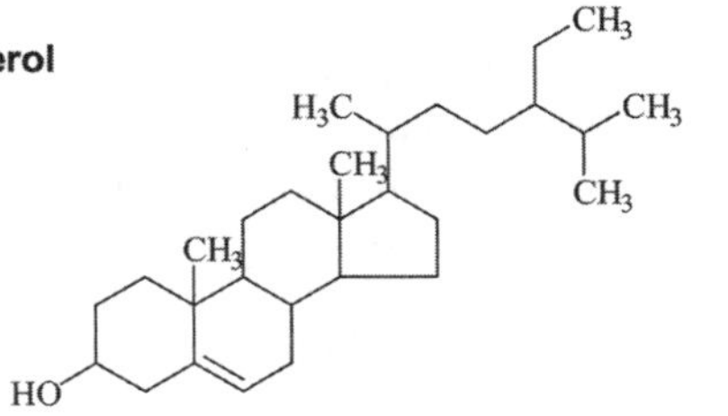

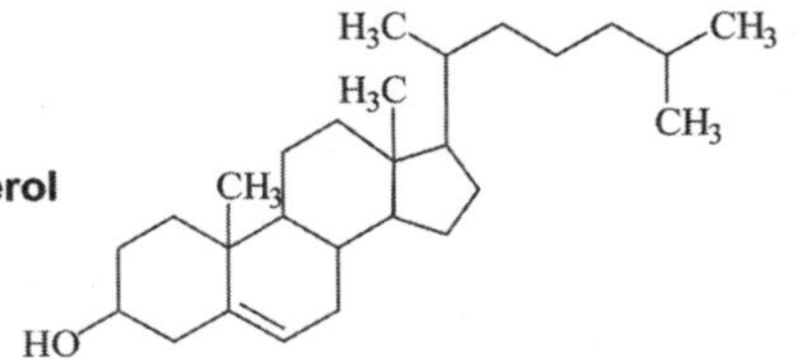

**Figure 2.10.** *The structural similarity between plant sterols like β-sitosterol and cholesterol results in molecular competition for intestinal absorption. Ancestral diets were rich in plant sterols and, hence, lower in cholesterol and its precursors.*

The angiotensin converting enzyme gene ACE I/D (insertion/deletion) polymorphism may be associated with salt-sensitive hypertension and it is certainly a candidate gene for the condition (65), although 20–30% of blood pressure variability is thought to stem from polygenes (66). An interesting hypothesis has been generated that suggests African-Americans may have inherited salt sensitivity from their slave ancestors, because individuals less resistant to salt loss died in transit across the Atlantic Ocean. Those with a genetic predisposition to retaining sodium were at an advantage, however, and survived the arduous sea voyage (67). Although this might explain why, among a hypertensive cohort, 76% of African-Americans were salt sensitive compared with only 56% of Caucasians (64,68), this hypothesis has been criticized on the basis of historical accounts that suggest salt may not have been limiting on these sea voyages (69). The likelihood of this particular hypothesis being correct is impossible to ascertain however; the advent of the agricultural revolution may have added selection pressures that worked on inherited salt sensitivity: Selection for salt sensitivity may have occurred due to the likely decline in hygiene conditions and the spread of diseases as a result of population aggregations associated with urbanization. In this scenario, it is possible that "thirsty" genes acted on sodium and water retention and aided survival from the stress of water volume depleting infectious diseases (64).

### 2.5.5 Balance between "Thrifty" and "Unthrifty" Alleles in Early Survival versus Late-Onset Diabetes

The curse of type 2 diabetes in modern cultures should not be taken for granted. In some populations the incidence of type 2 diabetes is extraordinarily high. On Nauru, a Pacific Micronesian island, in excess of 30% of islanders over 15 years of age have the disease.

These people have only recently begun to suffer from such high rates of type 2 diabetes, a condition virtually unknown at one time. Before the island's colonization by Britain and Australasia, the lives of islanders was extremely harsh, and an ability to rapidly build up fat at times of plenty in order to survive times of famine was very advantageous. The genes that permit this survival trait under ancestral conditions do not respond well to the typical Western diet. Nauru found prosperity through its guano deposits (bird droppings) that are hived off to fuel the world's need for phosphates. As a consequence of this newfound prosperity, islanders now have a far more sedentary lifestyle and calorie-rich diet that is out of synchrony with their ancestral genes and promotes the high incidence of type 2 diabetes. How significant are these "thrifty" genes on Nauru? Well, genes that were selected to confer advantage to islanders now represent the leading cause of nonaccidental death.

The so-called "thrifty genotype" hypothesis was actually first put forward to explain modern man's widespread susceptibility to type 2 diabetes. By default, one can postulate that allelic variants that offer protection against type 2 diabetes are "unthrifty" and have been the subject of selection pressures in the past (70).

The peroxisome proliferator-activated receptor-$\gamma$ (PPARG) nuclear receptor is critical for lipogenesis, energy metabolism, and insulin sensitivity. These multiple roles make it an important regulator of the "thrifty gene response" (71). The Ala12 variant of the PPARG gene (C1431T) has been linked to a diminished nuclear receptor activity, lower body mass index (BMI), and elevated insulin sensitivity compared with the Pro12 wildtype (72). It has been shown to be protective against type 2 diabetes in a range of ethnic groups (70). Thus, is the Ala12 variant an "unthrifty allele" of the PPARG gene that was exposed to negative selection during human evolution? Although difficult to evaluate, it has been deduced that data are compatible with neutrality of the Ala12 variant, and no evidence for negative selection has been found (70). However the same author does describe positive selection for this allele in an Indian population (70). Linkage disequilibrium estimates the age of the Ala12 variant to be around 27,000 years (70).

There is enormous interest in PPARG, largely because of its key role in lipogenesis, and as a direct consequence of its "master control" over the "thrifty gene response." Put simply, this receptor assists in efficient energy storage. This was great for our ancestors under the influence of a more primal diet, but bad for contemporary man. The role of PPARG in diabetes and obesity is of paramount importance, but it is also of interest because its synthetic ligands—thiazolidinediones—are promising insulin sensitizing drugs. PPARG is also crucial in transcriptional regulation of several cellular processes. These include control of the cell cycle, tumorigenesis, the inflammatory response, and immunomodulation (71,72).

## 2.6  THE EVOLUTION OF TASTE AS A SURVIVAL MECHANISM

The ability to taste and smell allows us to interact much more efficiently with our environment, and in the context of taste in particular, influences our choice of foods. Human taste can be broken down into five categories: salty, sour, sweet, umami, and bitter (73,74). The molecular basis of taste is similar to both smell and sight—see Figure 2.11.

It seems likely that the bitter modality may be especially important because it can alert us to many phytotoxins that tend to have a bitter taste. It is therefore reasonable to postulate that those humans with an acute sense of bitter taste may have had a better ability to survive in primitive environments (73,74).

# A brief account of the molecular mechanisms that underpin sight, olfaction, and gustation, key factors in optimal foraging

Efficiency in sequestering food was a likely determinant of survival for early man. His ability to taste (gustation), smell (olfaction), and see food (and predators) relied on similar but distinct sensory transduction mechanisms. Vision is of particular interest because it depends on dietary vitamin A as a light absorbing chromaphore (as 11-*cis*-retinal). 11-*cis*-retinal is covalently linked to a lysine residue on the opsin protein forming rhodopsin. When the vitamin A component of rhodopsin absorbs light, the photochemical energy converts 11-*cis*-retinal to all-*trans*-retinal. This biotransformation of the vitamin A chromaphore is the initial step in the visual transduction cycle that occurs in the rod and cone cells of the retina, and it is shown below in schematic form. Vitamin A deficiency is a huge global problem and can lead to permanent blindness.

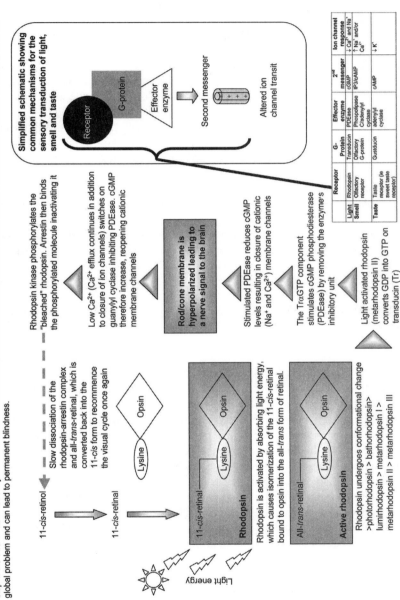

**Simplified schematic showing common mechanisms for the sensory transduction of light, smell and taste**

Second messenger

Altered ion channel transit

|  | Receptor | G-Protein | Effector enzyme | 2nd messenger | Ion channel response |
|---|---|---|---|---|---|
| Light | Rhodopsin | Transducin | PDEase | cGMP | ↓Ca²⁺ and Na⁺ |
| Smell | Olfactory receptor | Olfactory G-protein | Phospolipase C/adenylyl cyclase | IP3/cAMP | ↑Na and/or Ca²⁺ |
| Taste | Taste receptor (ie sweet taste receptor) | Gustducin | adenylyl cyclase | cAMP | ↓K⁺ |

Rhodopsin kinase phosphorylates the "bleached" rhodopsin. Arrestin then binds the phosphorylated molecule inactivating it

Low Ca²⁺ (Ca²⁺ efflux continues in addition to closure of ion channels) switches on guanylyl cyclase inhibiting PDEase. cGMP therefore increase, reopening cationic membrane channels

**Rod/cone membrane is hyperpolarized leading to a nerve signal to the brain**

Stimulated PDEase reduces cGMP levels resulting in closure of cationic (Na⁺ and Ca²⁺) membrane channels

The TrαGTP component stimulates cGMP phosphodiesterase (PDEase) by removing the enzyme's inhibitory unit

Light activated rhodopsin (metarhodopsin II) converts GDP into GTP on transducin (Tr)

Slow dissociation of the rhodopsin-arrestin complex and all-*trans*-retinal, which is converted back into the 11-*cis* form to recommence the visual cycle once again

11-*cis*-retinol

11-*cis*-retinal

11-*cis*-retinal — Lysine — Opsin

**Rhodopsin**

Rhodopsin is activated by absorbing light energy, which causes isomerization of the 11-*cis*-retinal bound to opsin into the all-*trans* form of retinal.

All-*trans*-retinal — Lysine — Opsin

**Active rhodopsin**

Rhodopsin undergoes conformational change >photorhodopsin > bathorhodopsin> lumirhodopsin > metarhodopsin I > metarhodopsin II > metarhodopsin III

Light energy

*Figure 2.11. A brief overview of the molecular signaling mechanisms that underpin sight, olfaction, and gustation, key factors in optimal foraging.*

Humans perceive bitterness as a consequence of signaling mediated by transmembrane G-protein-coupled receptors. The seven genes encoding these proteins are termed TAS2Rs or T2Rs. The genes are coexpressed in the taste receptor cells of the palate epithelium and tongue. Different receptors exhibit different substrate specificity, and this may explain why structurally diverse compounds are perceived to have a uniformly bitter taste (75).

Signatures of positive selection have been detected in one allelic form of the G-protein-coupled receptor encoded by TAS2R16, which mediates the signaling response to salicin, amygdalin, and a range of bitter $\beta$-glucopyranosides (74). Many $\beta$-glucopyranosides exhibit cyanogenic toxicity and are common plant constituents. Signatures of positive selection were detected in 997 individuals from 60 human populations as indicated by an excess of evolutionarily derived alleles at the nonsynonymous K172N site and two linked sites in 19 populations (74). The age that has been estimated for the origin of this trait to detect harmful cyanogenic glycosides is 78,700–791,000 years. This places its likely origins in the Middle Pleistocene and before early humans expanded out of Africa (74). These population studies were supported by intracellular signaling work using calcium imaging that showed N172 cells were associated with extra sensitivity to salicin, arbutin, and five different cyanogenic glycosides (74).

It would be difficult to argue against this selective event (conferred by the N172 allele) arising as an augmentation of fine control over ingestion of cyanogenic compounds. Compared with other mammalian species, humans have attenuated sensory traits; however, clearly preservation of specific sensory functions via positive selection was important in the earlier stages of human evolution (74) (see Figure 2.12).

## 2.7 THE MYSTERY OF ALCOHOL DEHYDROGENASE POLYMORPHISMS AND ETHANOL TOXICITY

Alcohol is removed from our circulation by the enzyme alcohol dehydrogenase (ADH), which converts it into acetaldehyde. Acetaldehyde is extremely toxic and, hence, is converted into acetyl CoA by acetaldehyde dehydrogenase (AcDH). Acetyl CoA is then delivered into either fatty acid metabolism or the tricarboxylic acid cycle.

A common East Asian genetic disposition exists, in which around half the population experience flushing around the face and neck due to high acetaldehyde levels after ingestion of alcohol. Such individuals have a variant form of ADH and an inefficient hepatic AcDH. This genetic trait may explain why early ancestors from this part of Asia relied on boiled water for safe potable beverages such as tea, whereas Europeans who can easily metabolize ethanol have historically relied on fermentation to produce safe drinking fluids.

Occurrence of the common ADH1B Arg47His polymorphism in Asians is a mystery: Why did selection of this seemingly deleterious allele occur? The ADH1B-47His allele has a very high frequency in the population that could not have occurred by random genetic drift alone (76). Selection must also have occurred, although this cannot be proven at this time. Consider also the AcDH protein, which acts as a dominant null allele that impairs the carrier's ability to degrade acetaldehyde. It is improbable that unlinked genes in two families in the same metabolic pathway that both increase toxic acetaldehyde could both have such high population frequencies by the random force of genetic drift alone. Although it is difficult to see how genetic drift could account for these two traits, it is equally difficult to explain their evolution in the context of natural selection (76). The causes behind the frequency of this unusual haplotype in East Asia remain a mystery.

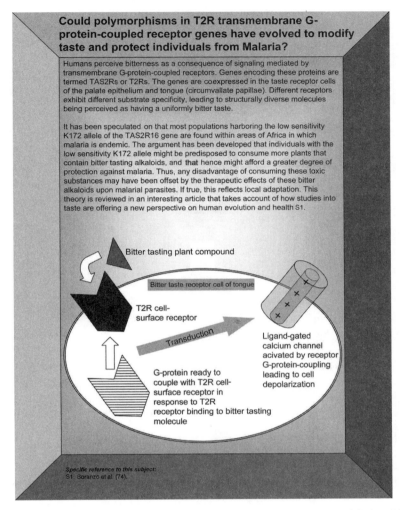

**Could polymorphisms in T2R transmembrane G-protein-coupled receptor genes have evolved to modify taste and protect individuals from Malaria?**

Humans perceive bitterness as a consequence of signaling mediated by transmembrane G-protein-coupled receptors. Genes encoding these proteins are termed TAS2Rs or T2Rs. The genes are coexpressed in the taste receptor cells of the palate epithelium and tongue (circumvallate papillae). Different receptors exhibit different substrate specificity, leading to structurally diverse molecules being perceived as having a uniformly bitter taste.

It has been speculated on that most populations harboring the low sensitivity K172 allele of the TAS2R16 gene are found within areas of Africa in which malaria is endemic. The argument has been developed that individuals with the low sensitivity K172 allele might be predisposed to consume more plants that contain bitter tasting alkaloids, and that hence might afford a greater degree of protection against malaria. Thus, any disadvantage of consuming these toxic substances may have been offset by the therapeutic effects of these bitter alkaloids upon malarial parasites. If true, this reflects local adaptation. This theory is reviewed in an interesting article that takes account of how studies into taste are offering a new perspective on human evolution and health S1.

Bitter tasting plant compound

Bitter taste receptor cell of tongue

T2R cell-surface receptor

Transduction

Ligand-gated calcium channel acivated by receptor G-protein-coupling leading to cell depolarization

G-protein ready to couple with T2R cell-surface receptor in response to T2R receptor binding to bitter tasting molecule

*Specific reference to this subject:*
S1. Soranzo et al. (74).

**Figure 2.12.** *Bitter taste may act to warn us against potentially toxic plants, but modulation of this sense via polymorphisms in the T2R transmembrane G-protein-coupled receptor genes could have evolved to protect individuals from Malaria.*

## 2.8 EVOLUTION OF XENOBIOTIC METABOLISM IN HUMANS

Xenobiotics are "foreign" chemicals that are not a normal component of the organism that is exposed to them. This includes most drugs and many plant phytochemicals that are alien to human metabolism, but that were nonetheless a part of our ancestral diet.

Humans have acquired the capability to avoid an accumulation of harmful dietary xenobiotics within cells as well as the ability to eliminate them from our bodies. To achieve this, multiple xenobiotic metabolizing enzymes with differential, but partly overlapping, catalytic properties assist in this elimination process (Figure 2.13).

These enzyme proteins, which are encoded by superfamilies of genes, have evolved in an adaptive manner that has made it possible for different species to survive and take

## Liver Metabolism of Xenobiotics

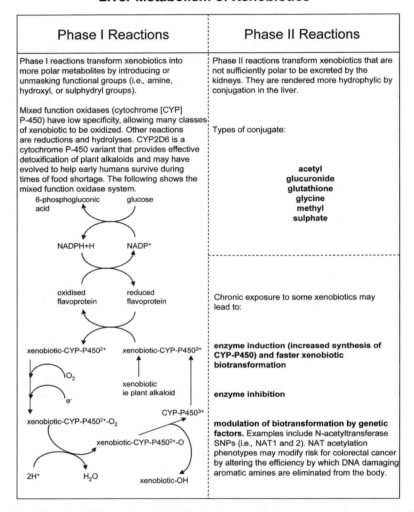

| Phase I Reactions | Phase II Reactions |
|---|---|
| Phase I reactions transform xenobiotics into more polar metabolites by introducing or unmasking functional groups (i.e., amine, hydroxyl, or sulphydryl groups). | Phase II reactions transform xenobiotics that are not sufficiently polar to be excreted by the kidneys. They are rendered more hydrophylic by conjugation in the liver. |

Mixed function oxidases (cytochrome [CYP] P-450) have low specificity, allowing many classes of xenobiotic to be oxidized. Other reactions are reductions and hydrolyses. CYP2D6 is a cytochrome P-450 variant that provides effective detoxification of plant alkaloids and may have evolved to help early humans survive during times of food shortage. The following shows the mixed function oxidase system.

Types of conjugate:

**acetyl**
**glucuronide**
**glutathione**
**glycine**
**methyl**
**sulphate**

Chronic exposure to some xenobiotics may lead to:

**enzyme induction (increased synthesis of CYP-P450) and faster xenobiotic biotransformation**

**enzyme inhibition**

**modulation of biotransformation by genetic factors.** Examples include N-acetyltransferase SNPs (i.e., NAT1 and 2). NAT acetylation phenotypes may modify risk for colorectal cancer by altering the efficiency by which DNA damaging aromatic amines are eliminated from the body.

**Figure 2.13.** *Phase I and II reactions in the liver help us to eliminate unnatural compounds from our body. Some polymorphisms of this system may help us better handle certain plant alkaloids that form an unwanted part of the diet and, hence, offer a survival advantage in particular environments.*

advantage of variable habitats and dietary patterns that exposes organisms to a variable level of potentially harmful alien chemicals. This evolutionary process has allowed species to develop xenobiotic metabolism unique to, and appropriate for, their survival.

This evolutionary process helps explain why inter-ethnic and inter-individual variability of drug metabolism exists in humans. As cancer-causing chemicals are substrates of drug-metabolizing enzymes, it is reasonable to assume that humans have a variable capacity to activate or inactivate carcinogens. Indeed, although most carcinogen-metabolizing enzymes are inducible by xenobiotics, they respond to environmental stimuli and thus can vary in activity; factors that influence activity include gender, age, circadian rhythm, liver disease, and other dietary components. Another source of variability germane to this treatise is that the genes that code for xenobiotic metabolizing enzymes can exist in polymorphic form, with multiple allelic variants determining the human phenotype for this detoxification process.

It therefore seems likely that genetic variability in the capacity to metabolize xenobiotics, including carcinogenic molecules, may be related to enzyme systems such as those involving cytochrome P450 (CYP450), glutathione S-transferase, and N-acetyltransferase gene families (77). As an example, polymorphic alleles carrying multiple active gene copies exist for CYP450 and, in the case of CYP2D6, are thought to be directed by positive selection due to development of alkaloid resistance by humans living in northeast Africa about 10,000–5000 BC (78). Although evolution has preserved CYP2D genes in rodents, inactivation has occurred in humans. Hence mice have nine active genes at this locus, but humans only have one. The human gene (CYP2D6) is polymorphic. The best explanation for this is that the rodent diet creates a greater need for inactivation of alkaloids than the human diet does. However, there are human exceptions. In northeast Africa, there has been selection for alleles containing multiple active copies of the CYP2D6 gene, such that up to 30% of individuals are affected in this way (78). The most plausible explanation for this is dietary selection. Individuals with more active copies of CYP2D6 would be more effective at detoxifying plant alkaloids and, thus, have a wider repertoire of food plants at their disposal during periods of potential starvation. This provides a putative advantage over individuals without "alkaloid resistance" (78).

Overall, 57 active CYP genes are known to be present in the human genome. To give a further idea of how useful isoforms of CYP are at dealing with foreign chemicals, CYP2C9, CYP2C19, CYP2D6, and CYP3A4 are particularly important for drug metabolism, whereas CYP1A1, CYP1A2, CYP1B1, CYP2E1, and CYP3A4 are critical for metabolic activation of precarcinogens (78). Not all isoforms, however, are associated with xenobiotic detoxification: CYP2R1 is active in the 25-hydroxylation of vitamin $D_2$ and $D_3$, but not for any known xenobiotic substrate, whereas CYP2U1 is preferentially expressed in the brain and metabolizes arachidonic acid.

Major allelic variants (SNPs) in these genes alter the efficacy of drugs, create side effects, and have specific impacts, such as on plant taxol metabolism. Interest in the variable ability of populations to biotransform xenobiotics extends beyond any ancestral advantage, and today, it occupies the realm of pharmacogenomics: how SNPs should be taken into account when ascertaining a drug's therapeutic efficacy and possible adverse reactions. See Figure 2.13 showing important biotransformation reactions.

Chapter *3*

# Essential Nutrients and Genomic Integrity: Developmental and Degenerative Correlates

It has been suggested that the DNA damage caused by a deficiency in any one of a large complement of minerals and vitamins can mimic the effect of radiation (79). That is, vitamins A, $B_{12}$, $B_6$, $B_3$, C, and E and folic acid along with zinc, magnesium, iron, and selenium are critical in preventing oxidative lesions and both single-and double-stranded DNA breaks (79) (Figure 3.1). They are also factors that can influence embryogenesis as well as being etiologically important in chronic adulthood diseases. Although the intricate relationship between folate and DNA damage has been described earlier, and is shown in Figures 2.8 and 2.9, the other vitamins are of similar relevance when considering the elaboration, maintenance, and expression of DNA (Table 3.1).

## 3.1 MICRONUTRIENTS AND GENOMIC STABILITY AND FUNCTION

### 3.1.1 Vitamin $B_{12}$

Vitamin $B_{12}$ deficiency is not uncommon and is a particular problem in the elderly where atrophic gastritis occurs. Reduced gastric juice pH and/or loss of intrinsic factor function diminish the bioavailability of this vitamin. As a consequence, folate is trapped at the level of 5-methyltetrahydrofolate because $B_{12}$-dependent methionine synthase activity is compromised (see Figure 2.9). This "functional folate deficiency" leads to a reduction in the

*Molecular Nutrition and Genomics: Nutrition and the Ascent of Humankind*, by Mark Lucock
Copyright © 2007 John Wiley & Sons, Inc.

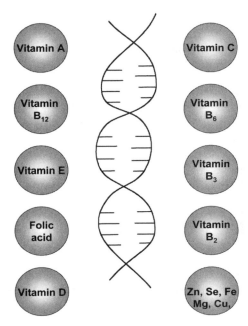

**Figure 3.1.** *Micronutrients that act directly or indirectly as antioxidants or influence DNA expression.*

folate vitamers required for dTMP synthesis and reduces the availability of *de novo* methyl groups required for CpG methylation and hence regulated DNA expression. The initial clinical manifestation of deficiency is an effect on red blood cells—megaloblastic anemia. This is a result of the secondary functional folate deficiency leading to uracil misincorporation in the developing erythroblasts. However, $B_{12}$ is also required for methylmalonylCoA-mutase, and deficiency at this locus can lead to failure to methylate an arginine residue on myelin basic protein and precipitate irreversible degeneration of the nervous system (see Figure 3.2). This "pernicious anemia" is very serious, and the early signs (megaloblastic anemia) are masked by excess intakes of folic acid—an argument often used against mandatory folate fortification policies. $B_{12}$ deficiency acts in synergy with folate deficiency to adversely affect DNA integrity, but studies have also identified a discrete influence of $B_{12}$ in this process (78).

### 3.1.2  Vitamin A

Retinoic acid (RA) interacts with receptors in the nucleus. RA binds to steroid and thyroid hormone receptors, which are a family of ligand-sensitive transcription factors. All-*trans* RA binds to the RA receptor (RAR), whereas 9-*cis* RA binds to the retinoid-X receptor (RXR). The binding of the heterodimer RAR/RXR to a specific "retinoic acid response element (RARE)" on DNA regulates gene transcription (Figure 3.3).

Vitamin A is probably best known for its role in vision (Figure 2.10) however, most of the physiological effects of vitamin A are a consequence of its hormone-like role in cellular differentiation; the morphogenetic properties of RA may stem from the activation of developmentally regulated genes by RA receptor (RAR) complexes. Indeed, women who

**Table 3.1. Important micronutrient–gene interactions, with particular reference to the effect of certain vitamins and minerals on the genomic machinery and/or gene product.**

| Some Important Micronutrient–Gene Interactions | | |
|---|---|---|
| Dietary Component | Background Information | Effect on Genomic Machinery and/or Gene Product |
| Retinoic acid (vitamin A) | RXR forms homodimers and heterodimers with vitamin D, PPAR, thyroid hormone, and COUP receptors | Binds either RXR or RAR nuclear retionoid receptor and enhances transcription, although in absence of retinoic acid, heterodimers repress gene expression |
| Ascorbic acid (vitamin C) | Oxidative DNA damage in vitamin C depletion (formation of 8-hydroxyguanine) | Enhances transcription of procollagen and translation of lysyloxidase |
| Pyridoxal Phosphate (vitamin $B_6$) | Modulates responsiveness of steroid hormone receptor | Attenuates transcription |
| Riboflavin (vitamin $B_2$) | Flavin cofactor for 5,10MTHFR | May interact with cellular folate to influence elaboration of DNA (1-C unit from folate donated to thymine) |
| Folic acid | Provides 1-C unit for purine, pyrimidine, and methyl groups | May modulate both expression of DNA via CpG methylation pattern and elaboration of DNA via provision of thymine. If 1-C shortage, uracil is misincorporated and DNA becomes unstable |
| Vitamin D | Vitamin D receptor forms a heterodimer with RXR | Enhances transcription of calcium binding proteins |
| Vitamin K | Growth arrest specific gene 6 product contains $\gamma$-carboxyglutamate residues | Regulates apoptosis, but it does not interact directly with genomic machinery |
| $\alpha$-Tocopherol (vitamin E) | Antioxidant properties. Ameliorates damage to DNA from excess iron. Induces two signal transduction pathways that act at several genes, but also acts independent of these two pathways | Protects genomic machinery from free radical damage. Alters activity of protein kinase C and phospotidylinositol 3-kinase. This in turn regulates the expression of several genes . Also acts on genes independent of these kinases |
| Calcium | Critical for intracellular signaling | Increased transcription of *c-fos*, *c-jun*, *c-myc* |
| Iron | During deficiency, iron-regulatory protein binds mRNA and promotes synthesis of transferrin receptor protein while ferritin production is repressed. The net effect is to increase iron utilization | Enhances transcription of metallothionein and translation of ferritin |
| Magnesium | Required for nucleic acid polymerase enzyme activity | Maintains fidelity of the DNA blueprint |
| Potassium | | Influences transcription of aldosterone synthase |
| Selenium | Selenocysteine residue in glutathione peroxidase provides antioxidant properties | Helps prevent free radical damage to genome |
| Zinc | Structural motif of zinc finger transcription factors | Augments transcription factor binding |

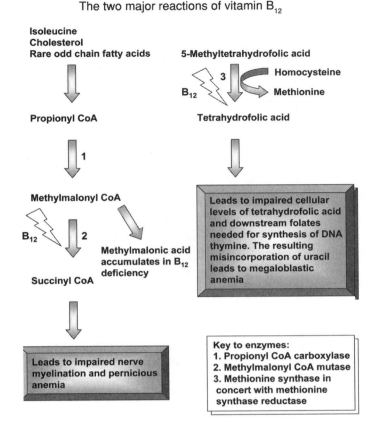

**Figure 3.2.** The role of vitamin $B_{12}$ in (1) preventing demyelination and pernicious anemia (methyl-malonyl CoA reaction) and (2) preventing megaloblastic anemia (methionine synthase reaction).

are pregnant or planning a pregnancy should limit their intake of vitamin A to avoid the potential for birth defects as this vitamin, and its pharmacologic analogs, are considered to be teratogenic.

Vitamin A is of two types—preformed and provitamin A. Provitamin A types represent the polyphenolic carotenoids, and include $\alpha$-carotene, $\beta$-carotene, $\gamma$-carotene, and $\beta$-cryptoxanthine (Figure 3.4). $\beta$-carotene in particular has an important role as a free radical scavenger, and it protects DNA and membrane structures when present at an appropriate level. As this molecule is obtained from plant sources, an individual with good levels of $\beta$-carotene is also likely to have a healthy level of many other phytonutrients that benefit the structure and function of the cell.

### 3.1.3 Vitamin $B_2$

A synergy is likely to exist between riboflavin and folic acid. Supplementation with vitamin $B_2$ may improve the activity of the variant form of C677T-MTHFR and, therefore, improve folate-dependent pathways such as *de novo* methionine biosynthesis needed to maintain

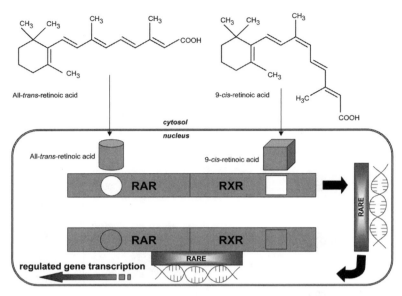

**Figure 3.3.** Schematic of vitamin A and gene regulation.

genomic CpG methylation patterns, as well as regeneration of tetrahydrofolate for nucleotide biosynthesis. This is because MTHFR is a flavoprotein.

### 3.1.4 Vitamin B$_6$

B$_6$ along with B$_{12}$ and folate help to regulate the methionine cycle and the balance between homocysteine remethylation and its transulphuration to cysteine. Cystathionine $\beta$-synthase and $\gamma$-cystathionase are both transulphuration pathway enzymes and both B$_6$ dependent. Homocysteine is thought to be embryotoxic, and thus, dietary B$_6$, B$_{12}$, and folate may critically influence the level of homocysteine exposed to the early embryo, impacting on reproductive success.

B$_6$ is also important in the regulation of steroid hormones, because it helps to remove the hormone-receptor complex from DNA binding and, hence, terminates hormone action. Hence, when B$_6$ is deficient, there is an increased sensitivity to circulating hormone levels.

### 3.1.5 Vitamin B$_3$

The transfer of ADP-ribose moieties from B$_3$ (niacin) derived NAD to arginine, lysine, or asparagine residues of nucleoproteins involved in DNA repair and replication is catalyzed by poly-ADP-ribose polymerases (PARPs). Five or more different PARPs exist, and in the region of a double-strand DNA break, hundreds of ADP-ribose molecules are polymerized per minute. It is therefore not surprising that a deficiency of vitamin B$_3$ leads to DNA instability.

# Biologically important antioxidant carotenoids

α-Carotene

β-Carotene

Cryptoxanthin

Lycopene

Zeaxanthin

Lutein

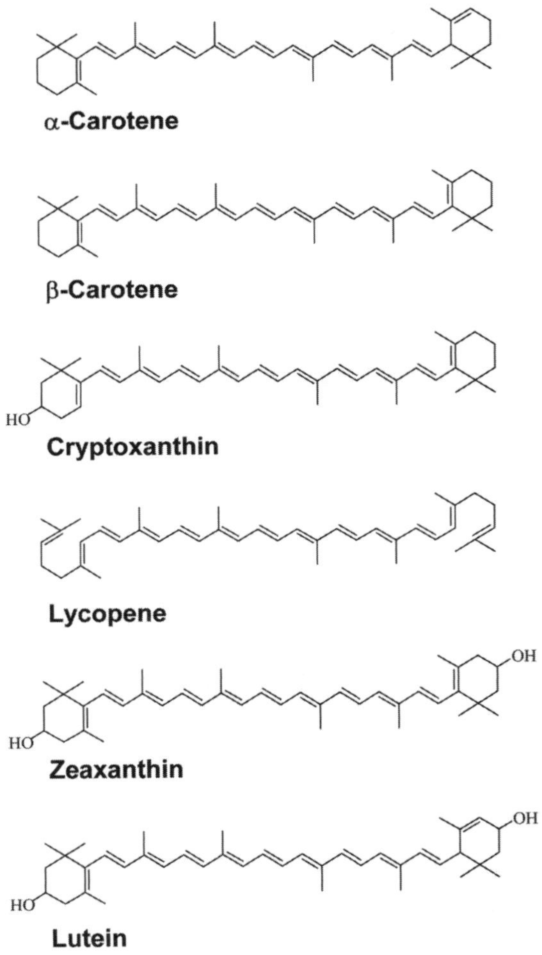

**Figure 3.4.** *Figure showing the biologically important antioxidant carotenoids. β-Carotene status reflects a diet rich in fruit and vegetables and is an important cellular antioxidant, although it can also act as a pro-oxidant in excess. It also acts as a provitamin A nutrient, providing the body with this essential fat-soluble vitamin after intestinal hydrolysis by carotene dioxygenase. Lutein is concentrated in the macular of the eye, where it protects the retina by neutralizing free radicals. Lycopene is a potent antioxidant found in tomato products and is thought to protect cells against malignant change. Carotenoids are considered to be extremely beneficial nutrients with substantial health benefits.*

## 3.1.6   Antioxidant Micronutrients (Vitamins E, C, β-carotene, and Selenium)

A deficiency in these important antioxidant nutrients will cause chromosomal damage and oxidative lesions to membrane structures.

Outside of its crucial role as a coenzyme for copper-dependent hydroxylases and α-ketoglutarate-linked iron-containing hydroxylases, vitamin C has generalized antioxidant properties, including salvage of the spent tocopheroxyl radical back to α-tocopherol (vitamin

E). Vitamin C can neutralize reactive oxygen species (ROS) and, hence, protect nuclear and membrane structures:

It is worth noting that at high levels, vitamin C, as with other antioxidants such as $\beta$-carotene, may actually potentiate radical formation and compromise the integrity of genomic mechanisms (see carotenoid Figure 3.4 above):

### Vitamin C as a protective antioxidant:

ascorbate + $^\bullet O_2^-$ + $H^+$ → $H_2O_2$ + monodehydroascorbate (stable, and salvageable vitamin C radical)

### Vitamin C as a prooxidant source of free radicals:

ascorbate + $O_2$ → $^\bullet O_2^-$ + monodehydroascorbate

Monodehydroascorbate can be enzymatically returned to ascorbate via monodehydroascorbate reductase or undergo dismutation to ascorbate and dehydroascorbate (see Figure 3.5).

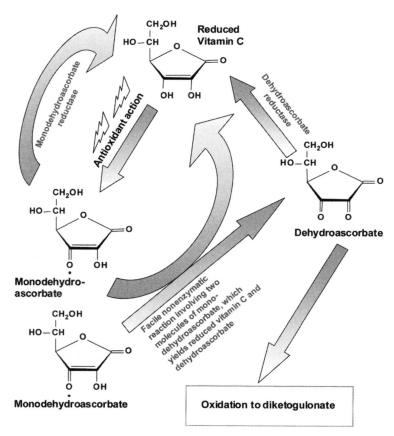

**Figure 3.5.** Scheme showing antioxidant effect and salvage of vitamin C.

Haptoglobin polymorphisms are associated with inflammatory and immune diseases possibly due to a phenotype-dependent modulation of oxidative stress and prostaglandin synthesis. Strong genetic selection favors the HP2-2 phenotype indicating an important role of haptoglobin in human pathology.

Haptoglobin is an acute-phase plasma protein that binds free hemoglobin and thus prevents catalysis of reactive oxygen species. The HP2-2 phenotype of the haptoglobin gene leads to an accumulation of iron, making individuals more susceptible to disease by lowering vitamin C levels. In other words, a higher rate of L-ascorbic acid oxidation in Hp2-2 carriers occurs because they have less protection against hemoglobin–iron-driven peroxidation (80, 81). This vitamin C-related gene–nutrient interaction might well be a significant one in determining evolutionary fitness. It is interesting to consider that lower levels of potentially prooxidant vitamin C at the onset of infection may actually protect tissue from excessive free radical damage via mechanisms such as the macrophage respiratory burst.

Vitamin E protects polyunsaturated fatty acids within the cell membrane and plasma lipoproteins from lipid peroxidation. It reduces lipid peroxide radicals to unreactive fatty acids. As a consequence of peroxyl-radical scavenging, vitamin E is converted into the stable tocopheroxyl radical. Both vitamin C and the selenium enzyme glutathione peroxidase can salvage this compound back into $\alpha$-tocopherol. It is this role that classifies selenium as an antioxidant (Figures 2.7, 3.5, and 3.6 show the salvage mechanisms for important native antioxidant micronutrients). See earlier for significance in gametogenesis.

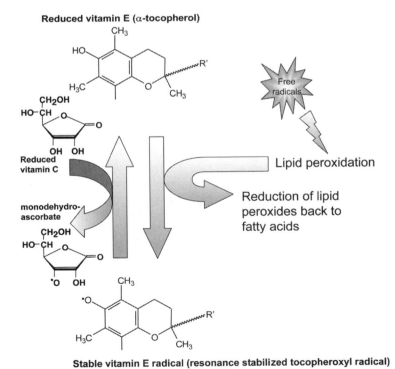

**Figure 3.6.** *Vitamin E ($\alpha$-tocopherol) can reduce lipid peroxides but in the process becomes oxidized. Vitamin C reduces the relatively stable tocopheroxyl radical back to $\alpha$-tocopherol.*

$\alpha$-Tocopherol also modulates two important signal transduction pathways that are centered on phospatidylinositol 3-kinase and protein kinase C. These pathways alter cell proliferation, platelet aggregation, and NADPH-oxidase activation. $\alpha$-Tocopherol also regulates genes independent of these kinase pathways. $\gamma$-Tocopherol also has some gene regulatory properties (82).

### 3.1.7  Vitamin D

Calcitriol (vitamin $D_3$) is the active form of vitamin D and elicits an effect on gene transcription via the vitamin D receptor (VDR), which forms a heterodimer with the RXR (retinoid-X receptor). Thus, vitamins A and D work in concert for many genomic-functions of vitamin D. Polymorphisms of the VDR (Figure 3.7) may act by a similar gene–nutrient interaction to that of the MTHFR SNP in respect to the etiology of human disease (25): Vitamin $D_3$ is thought to protect against breast cancer. VDR polymorphisms are associated with breast cancer risk and may be associated with disease progression. It is thought that VDR polymorphisms modulate the interaction between $D_3$ and the VDR gene product and that they could lead to a differential responsiveness of target cells to the action of $D_3$ (83).

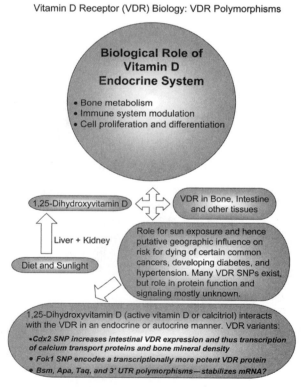

**Figure 3.7.** Vitamin D receptor (VDR) biology plays an important role in bone metabolism, immune system function, and cell growth and differentiation: Polymorphisms exist in the VDR and influence such things as calcium transport and bone mineral density.

## 3.1.8 Zinc, Manganese, Magnesium, Iron, and Copper

Zinc has a wide range of effects within a panoply of dependent proteins, many of which are tasked with maintaining replication and the normal functioning of DNA. Examples include "zinc finger proteins," which act as important transcription factors. Zinc is present at vastly elevated levels in seminal fluid compared with blood plasma. This implies a critical role for zinc in spermatogenesis and spermatozoal stability (84). Low zinc levels are found in infertile males and are associated with increased damage to testicular DNA (85). Magnesium is equally important. This essential cation maintains the fidelity of DNA transcription. By contrast, iron may actually cause chromosomal damage in excess or deficiency. Vitamin E is thought to ameliorate this effect. During iron deficiency, iron-regulatory protein binds mRNA and promotes synthesis of transferrin receptor protein while ferritin production is repressed. The net effect is to increase iron utilization.

Metal ions such as copper and iron are catalysts in the degradation of peroxides and, hence, can cause the formation of the DNA and membrane damaging $^{\bullet}OH$ free radical (see below for full account of free radical biochemistry). For this reason, metal ion–protein binding complexes evolved. Initially, they will not have inactivated the catalytic redox potential of metal ions but simply diverted deleterious free radicals away from nuclear material and membrane structures (86). This kind of protective mechanism by proteins, in which radical damage is targeted on the protein ligand itself in a kamikaze-like manner, is still observed today: Albumin is an example of a protein that can act as a sacrificial antioxidant buffer (86). However, more effective strategies have evolved to permit inactivation of the copper and iron catalytic redox potential: Specific proteins such as ceruloplasmin (carries $Cu^{2+}$), ferritin, and transferrin (carry $Fe^{3+}$) emerged. These proteins maintain free iron and copper at levels that minimize catalytic formation of $^{\bullet}OH$ (86–88).

As peroxides are deleterious and generate $^{\bullet}OH$, catalases and peroxidases have evolved in eukaryotes to remove hydrogen peroxide. Most of these beneficial antioxidant enzymes contain $Fe^{3+}$ protoporphyrin at their catalytic site. Natural selection has evolved an elegant cooperativity among enzyme systems to turn toxic hydrogen peroxide into water, and the localization of this noxious substance and catalase activity to specialized structures within the cell known as peroxisomes (catalase step; $2H_2O_2 \rightarrow 2H_2O + O_2$).

It is interesting that heme iron is absorbed around five times more efficiently than is inorganic iron obtained from vegetables and grain. This fact implies the existence of a transporter of heme iron from the gut into intestinal mucosal cells. This long sought after transporter has recently been found (89), and is designated HCP1. Duodenal HCP1 shifts position within intestinal mucosal cells in response to changes in the body's iron stores, allowing cells to take up more, or less, heme iron as required. This protein will be an interesting target for both genetic and pharmacologic research over coming years. Examples of potential benefits include improved synthetic analogs of heme iron that are better tolerated and more readily absorbed, and better therapies for hemochromatosis sufferers.

One of the most important enzymes that counter free radical damage alongside catalase and peroxidase is superoxide dismutase, often referred to as SOD (catalyses; $^{\bullet}O_2^- + H_2O \rightarrow 2H_2O_2 + O_2$). Two intracellular forms of SOD exist in mammals: a mitochondrial, tetrameric manganese-containing enzyme and a cytosolic, dimeric copper/zinc-containing enzyme. The importance of these enzymes highlights once again the significance of these metal ion ligands. The Cu, Zn-SODs have been shown to have underwent Darwinian natural selection, and exhibit significant changes in evolutionary rate, with accelerated evolution in both great apes and humans. These findings are inconsistent with the neutral theory of genetic drift and demonstrate clear selection. By contrast, Mn-SODs seem to have evolved at a far more constant rate (90).

One can unite these critically important antioxidant enzyme systems into a singular process that helps neutralize radicals such as the superoxide radical as shown:

SOD reaction:

$$^\bullet O_2^- + H_2O \rightarrow O_2 + 2H_2O_2$$

Catalase/peroxidase reaction:

$$H_2O_2 \rightarrow 2H_2O + O_2$$

The intimate association of so many essential dietary micronutrients with the genomic machinery explains why there is so much clinical interest in these molecules at the beginning and end of the human lifecycle. Furthermore, it would be unsurprising if these dietary components did not, in some small way, help to fashion our ancestral lineage.

# Chapter 4

# Nutrients and Cerebral Function in Human Evolution

## 4.1 HUMAN ENCEPHALISATION MAY BE LINKED TO AN EVOLUTIONARY REDUCTION IN GUT MASS

Humans are unusual in that they have a larger brain size than might be predicted based on their body size. Such dramatic encephalization has only occurred in the last 2–3 million years, with a three-fold increase in brain size since the time of *Australopithecus aferensis* (the "Lucy" skeleton) 4.5 million years ago (91). To permit this degree of encephalization, two requirements must have been met: (1) adequate supply of polyunsaturated fatty acids, in particular, arachidonic and docosahexaenoic acids and (2) an increase in cerebral metabolic capacity (92–95). It has been suggested that the availability of these fatty acids may have acted as a selective pressure driving encephalization, simply by provision of an adequate dietary substrate (96,97).

A large brain mass comes at a cost: the metabolic price for cerebral maintenance being nine-fold higher than that for the body as a whole (97). To sustain a large brain, an evolutionary adaptation may have been made. It is believed that a surplus in cerebral mass and energy need is closely counterbalanced by a reduction in the mass and associated energy needs of the gastrointestinal tract (97). Indeed, the relationship between body size and gut size are clearly linked via diet; herbivores, which eat bulky, macronutrient poor foods have large complex guts, whereas carnivores that eat a less bulky nutrient-dense diet have smaller, simple stomachs with a long intestine but smaller colon. The trend among primates is toward a high-quality diet, small gut, and large brain, with humans having an extremely high encephalization quotient of 4.6 based on the Martin equation (91,97). This encephalization quotient has probably been achieved by a move toward a meat-based diet rich in unsaturated fats. Indeed, Mann (91) has suggested that our consumption of a diet much higher in quality than expected for our size is an adaptation to the high metabolic needs of our large brain, and that this encephalization is a trade off against gut size.

An interesting line of enquiry suggests that what differentiates modern humans from the great apes and Neanderthals are genes coding for proteins that control fat metabolism, and in particular regulation of the phospholipid metabolism of brain synapses (98). It has been suggested that between 7 and 0.6 million years ago, the genomic machinery related to the efficiency of fat uptake into tissues, and the phospholipid-associated organization of synapses led to a slow growth of brain size. However, from 150,000 years ago, a rapid growth of brain size and attendant cognitive and memory skills developed. This, it is suggested, arose due to a key mutation(s) in phospholipid metabolism akin to that observed in the Mensa mouse and Dougie mouse (genetically engineered smart super-mice). The contention is that little change occurred to the number of nerve cells, while much more complex connections formed. The key mutation(s) that helped propel human intellect may have taken place 150,000–130,000 years ago in our immediate ancestor, but not Neanderthals, and could well have been related to the phospholipase $A_2$ cycle (98). Although this postulate could account for amplified cognitive flexibility, creativity, and inventiveness through a link between dietary fat and phospolipid-related brain anatomy, these mutations may also conspire with dietary deficits in the range and quantity of essential fatty acids needed by the brain, to create neuro-psychiatric disorders like schizophrenia (98).

Non-nutritional effects are also likely to be crucial: The abnormal spindle-like microcephaly associated (ASPM) gene produces a functional protein that has an unclear role in brain, although it is associated with an abnormal mitotic spindle apparatus, causing *Drosophila* neuroblasts to arrest in metaphase. Evolutionary selection of specific segments of the ASPM gene sequence strongly relates to primate cerebral cortical size (99,100). Another hypothesis suggests that human intelligence and brain development evolved in relation to thyroid and steroid hormone metabolism (101).

Evolutionary biologists put particular emphasis on genes implicated in microcephaly, and they propose that a subset of these genes have played a role in brain enlargement over time. ASPM is such a gene as are MCPH1 and SHH (102).

Clearly, many factors are likely to have conspired in the process of human encephalization—some with a clear nutritional basis, some, such as the putative adaptive evolution of ASPM being consistent with the evolutionary enlargement of the human brain, less so.

## 4.2 WEANING AND BRAIN DEVELOPMENT

Human infants are dependent on their parents for longer than any other hominoid. Nevertheless, *Homo sapiens* are actually weaned much earlier (by on average 2.5 years) than the young of contemporary great apes. Kennedy (103) has sought an explanation for this divergence in human weaning patterns from those of other hominoids, particularly given the hazards of early weaning.

Kennedy (103) contends that if selection favored the survival of the child, human infants would suckle as long as their hominoid relatives (weaning deprives the infant of maternal milk-immune factors and exposes an immature gut and dentition to an adult food supply). As a consequence, this author suggests that selection favors some trait other than the child's survival. Kennedy argues that developmentally early brain growth, which is the neurological basis of our intellectual ability, cannot be sustained by lactation beyond the first year of life. Therefore, early weaning and the attendant consumption of more nutritious foods of animal origin provide an evolutionary focus on intellectual development as a selective trait over infant survival.

This paradigm could have been shaped by a shift from hunted prey to utilization of carcasses concomitant with the use of primitive tools for butchery. This approach facilitated an increase in calories and protein irrespective of habitat. This form of foraging may have lead to direct competition with carnivorous mammals leading to the socioevolutionary adaptation of alloparenting. These subtle changes in diet are therefore putative drivers of brain development and hence quite possibly significant factors in the origins of the genus *Homo* (103).

Figure 4.1 shows the changing dimension of certain human structures. Of particular significance is the increase in brain size and the consequent need for a high-quality diet to maintain cerebral metabolic needs. This growth may have been driven by complex environmental and social factors, as well as by key genetic mutations.

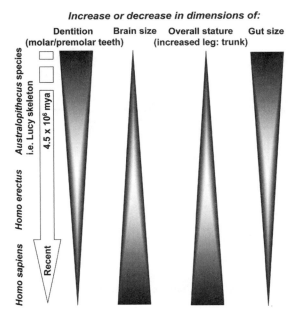

**Figure 4.1.** *Dramatic encephalization has only occurred in the last 2–3 million years, with a three-fold increase in brain size since the time of* Australopithecus aferensis *(the "Lucy" skeleton) 4.5 million years ago. A diet much higher in quality than expected for our size may be an adaptation to the high metabolic needs of our large brain, and this encephalization could thus be a trade off against gut size. Key mutation(s) that helped propel human intellect have occurred recently, including nonnutritional ones like ASPM, MCPH1, and SHH. Human accelerated region1 (HAR1), a noncoding DNA sequence producing RNA in Cajal-Retzius cells in the brain, evolved so rapidly in humans that this may be what made us different from other primates. So it may be that noncoding DNA rather than protein coding sequences have rewired the brain to human specifications. Clearly, we still have much to learn about our origins.*

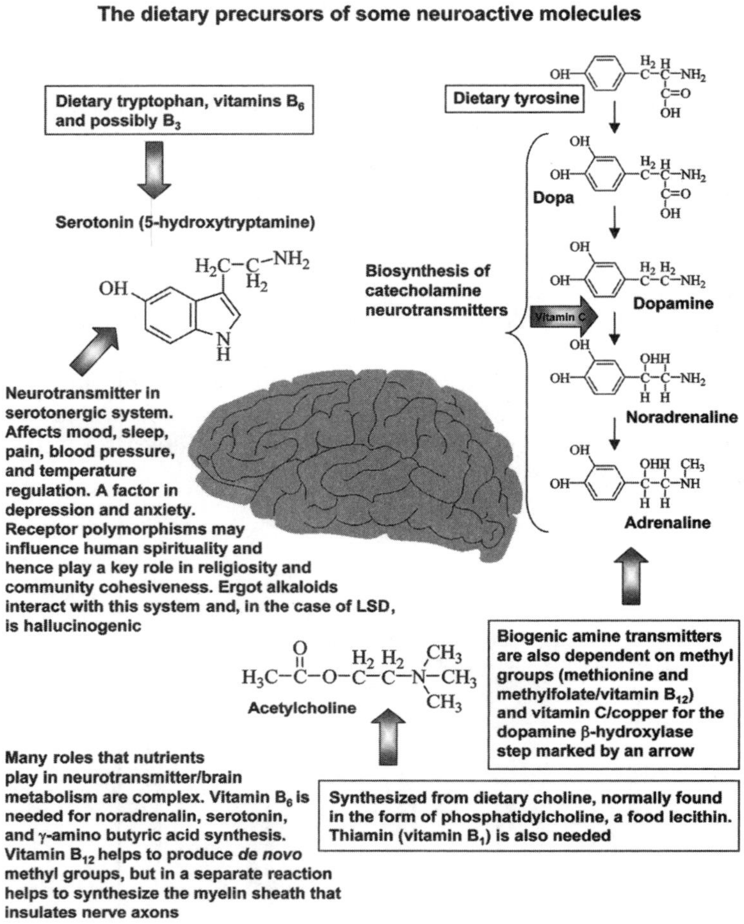

**The dietary precursors of some neuroactive molecules**

*Figure 4.2.* The corollary between certain key dietary nutrients and brain neurotransmitter metabolism.

## 4.3 MICRONUTRIENTS AND THE CEREBRAL BASIS OF SPIRITUALITY AND SOCIAL STRUCTURE

At a more subtle level, several individual micronutrients that are dietary essentials play a fundamental role in brain development and function and, via common polymorphisms in neuronal proteins, likely influence behavioral traits that contribute to human social structure.

An important brain-nutrient relationship is represented by s-adenosylmethionine (SAM) produced *de novo* from 5-methyltetrahydrofolate and vitamin $B_{12}$, or originated directly from dietary methionine. SAM is the methyl donor for several methylation reactions involving biogenic amine (monoamine neurotransmitter) metabolism. Reactions involve catechol-O-methyltransferase, hydroxyindole-O-methyltransferase, and phenylethanolamine-N-methyltransferase, all of which are crucial for the synthesis of neuronal products (23,104). Modulation of this area of neurotransmitter metabolism is thought to impact on mood due to the altered monoamine level in the region of the synapse—indeed folate levels have long been associated with affective disorders (105). However, this kind of pharmacology may be implicated in a much more subtle sociogenomic interaction that has modulated the social evolution of man. The complex personality trait best referred to as "spirituality" is thought to be influenced by several genes in tandem with environmental factors. This trait is assessed using the Temperament and Character Inventory to yield an index of self-transcendence, which includes measures of openness to things not literally provable, connectedness to a larger universe, and an ability to get lost in an experience. The vesicular monoamine transporter-2 gene (VMAT2) encodes a protein that controls the transport of monoamine neurotransmitters. It has been postulated that polymorphic forms of this gene may well account for a part of the observed variability in spirituality that exists (106). It has been suggested that by individuals evolving a sense of spirituality, society as a whole thrived. Two lines of research into indoleamine monoamine transmitter metabolism further support this paradigm and suggest a role for a variant of the $5\text{-HT}_{1A}$ gene (C-to-G substitution at position 92928) encoding the serotonin 1A receptor in human spiritual inclinations (107). A direct role for SAM produced *de novo* from 5-methyltetrahydrofolate and $B_{12}$ in the synthesis of catecholamine monoamine neurotransmitters is beyond doubt. However, there is also speculation that a direct transfer of methyl groups from 5-methyltetrahydrofolate to both indole- and catecholamine monoamines may occur to form tetrahydro-$\beta$-carboline derivatives independent of SAM. Tetrahydro-$\beta$-carboline derivatives are potent inhibitors of the neuronal uptake of 5-hydroxytryptamine (5-HT/serotonin), dopamine, and noradrenaline, and of the deamination of 5-HT (104). This finding adds potential weight to a paradigm in which micronutrients may have played an important role in both the content and the expression of our cerebral being. Although tetrahydro-$\beta$-carboline psychotogens are formed *in vitro* directly from folate without the mediation of SAM, their presence *in vivo* remains to be proven. However, there is little doubt that as well as being a source of methyl groups for biogenic amine synthesis, folate is directly required for the synthesis of the inhibitory transmitter glycine (108), and that it modifies the uptake of neurotransmitters into the nerve endings (109). Furthermore, several reports also indicate a degree of metabolic overlap between folate and biopterin pathways due to the commonality of the pterin; 2-amino-4-hydroxypteridine, in both molecular structures. This is important because aromatic amino acid hydroxylases such as tyrosine hydroxylase use biopterin for synthesis of DOPA and downstream biogenic amines from tyrosine (see Figures 2.6 and 4.1) (110,111). It has been suggested that folate may also interact directly with neuronal membrane receptors (112,113).

Perhaps less significant, but worthy of note, dietary sources of vitamin $B_3$ (niacin) are augmented by endogenous formation of NAD from tryptophan, a process that is also dependent on adequate vitamin $B_6$ due to $B_6$ being a cofactor for kynureninase. Dietary tryptophan is a more important source of NAD than are preformed dietary sources of the vitamin and is the precursor of 5-HT in the central nervous system (CNS). In Hartnup disease, for instance, impaired uptake of tryptophan leads not only to a deficit of 5-HT, but also it leads to pellagra, the vitamin $B_3$ deficiency disease.

An interactive combination of known and yet-to-be-discovered complex cerebral phenomena such as serotonin 1A receptor density (114) and the $5\text{-HT}_{1A}$ and VMAT2 gene variants (106,107) may well have played a critical role in the development of a common system of beliefs and practices that underpin secular rules that maintain the day-to-day functioning of a population group. A possible mechanistic role for micronutrients in the evolution of this process cannot be ignored. Folate, $B_3$, $B_6$, and $B_{12}$ have been discussed; however, the role of vitamins A, C, $B_1$, and a second role for $B_{12}$ and $B_6$

should also be mentioned. Vitamin A regulates gene expression and cell differentiation and turnover.

As part of vitamin A developmental regulation, neuronal malformations have been noted. Vitamin C is required for dopamine-$\beta$-hydroxylase. This enzyme is needed for the biosynthesis of the biogenic amine noradrenaline from tyrosine in the CNS. Dopamine-$\beta$-hydroxylase requires $Cu^+$, which is oxidized to $Cu^{2+}$ during hydroxylation. Reduction back to $Cu^+$ creates an obligate need for vitamin C. Vitamin $B_{12}$ is needed by methylmalonyl-CoA mutase for synthesis of brain myelin, whereas vitamin $B_6$ is crucial for the synthesis of many neurotransmitters such as $\gamma$-aminobutyric acid (GABA), noradrenaline, and 5-HT. Deficiency can lead to depression, confusion, and even convulsions. Vitamin $B_1$ (thiamin) is important in the synthesis of acetylcholine, another neurotransmitter, and may be important in ion translocation within neurons. The essential nature of these "food constituents" as potentially important environmental factors in evolutionary processes should not be over-looked. Clearly, the potential for several gene–nutrient interactions in the evolution of our cerebral being is a distinct possibility.

## 4.4 PHARMACOTOXICOLOGY OF PLANTS AND CULTURAL EVOLUTION

There are two facets to the pharmacotoxicology of plants and our cultural evolution that I will discuss here. One is more a point of interest that leads on to issues of relevance; the other is a deeper issue that has impacted on many societies, both old and new.

Ancient writings make note of a corollary between the consumption of certain grains and sometimes bizarre human diseases. Sacred writing from 2500 years ago refers to the toxicity of grasses that acted as agents leading to the death of pregnant women and/or their fetuses. Romans, in the first century BC reported that grain spoilage was the cause of epidemics that persisted as a regular occurrence up to the Middle Ages in European countries. However, it was not until the seventeenth century that a clear relationship was established between spoiled grain contaminated with the fungus *Claviceps prupurea* and ergotism. Today we know that when grain becomes moist under the right conditions, the germination of up to 50 species of *Claviceps* (ergot) can occur, and all are capable of causing ergotism.

There are two types of ergot poisoning. The first type is gangrenous poisoning, which is associated with severe pain, along with a burnt and inflamed appearance to the limbs, which in the worst cases turn black. The appearance of afflicted individuals is as if they were burned. As a result, ergotism had the alternative name "Holy Fire". The pharmacologic basis of this is vasoconstriction resulting from the ergot stimulating effect on smooth muscle. The second form of ergotism is referred to as convulsive ergotism, and it is less well understood. The effects are numbness, paralysis, loss of sight, and convulsions. The neurological basis of this form has been variously linked to nutritional status, genetic variation of afflicted people, and neuroactive substances from other fungi present with *Claviceps*. It has also been suggested that women implicated as witches during the Salem Witch Trials in the late 1600s may have been suffering the effects of eating ergot-infected rye bread. By 1692, 20 people had been put to death in Massachusetts for their crimes. All of the accused had similar symptoms: manic depression, delirium, psychosis, crawling sensations within the skin, vertigo, headaches, and gastrointestinal upsets. All of which are symptoms of ergot poisoning. In an interesting *Science* article (115), it has been postulated that the Salem Witch Trials coincided with a weather period that would have produced large quantities of *C. purpurea* ergot on the locally grown rye.

The principle bioactive of ergot is a family of lysergic-acid-type alkaloids. Today these alkaloids (ergotoxin, ergonovine, and ergotamine) have all found a prominent therapeutic role in modern medicine. However, it is perhaps molecules like the synthetic amide derivative of lysergic acid, i.e., LSD, that act as potent hallucinogens, which are of most significance in human cultural evolution. Indeed, hallucinogens have had a long and varied role in human societies.

Entheogens (literally translated to mean that which causes a person to be in God) are age-old drugs derived from natural products (mescalin from peyote cactus [*Lophophora wiliamsii*], psilocybin from certain mushrooms [magic mushrooms are familiar to many of us in the West, *Psilocybe aztecorum* was the narcotic mushroom used by Aztec society]) that cause people to have metaphysical experiences. In many cases, these drugs act at the pharmacological sites mentioned above (serotonergic neuronal circuits, for example, are where LSD acts). As contended, this kind of pharmacogenomics (genetic polymorphisms in catechol and indoleamine neurotransmitter metabolism) seems to be implicated in a subtle sociogenomic interaction that may have impacted on the social evolution of man because modulation of the neuronal circuits encoded by our genes lead to religious tendencies. Shamans have exploited this phenomenon for thousands of years. As an example, the Apaches of the Great Plains developed a religious peyote rite.

These molecules originate from plants, but their categorization as foods is somewhat tenuous. One could argue the case that they were a minor element within the diets of certain societies. Strictly speaking, they are psychotomimetics, hallucinogenics, or psychedelics.

The science of pharmacology contains many similar anecdotes, many of which have some passing relevance to the nature of this thesis. Centuries-old practices have aided the functioning of societies, eking out an existence in difficult environments. For example, in the foothills of the Himalayas, *Rauwolfia serpentina* was used as a sedative. The bioactive constituent, reserpine, had a calming effect on patients with mental and physical disorders and was used wherever appropriate, such as for example to treat the panic after snakebite envenomation. The analgesic value of morphine-like compounds needs little explanation. In 1680, referring to the various morphine alkaloids derived from *Papaver somniferum*, Syndenham wrote that "Among the remedies which it has pleased Almighty God to give to man to relieve his sufferings, none is so universal and so efficacious as opium." The benefits of plant medicines in the context of social evolution is a subject that deserves an entire volume devoted to it, and it is beyond the scope to be covered here.

Chapter *5*

# The Evolution of Micronutrient Metabolism

## 5.1 ANTIOXIDANTS, EVOLUTION, AND HUMAN HEALTH

One of the great biological paradoxes is that although oxygen is vital for much planetary life, it can also cause great damage to our delicate cellular mechanisms. Antioxidant mechanisms therefore evolved to cope with the rise of an oxygen-rich atmosphere (Figure 5.1). A diet rich in plant antioxidants augments our inherent defense strategies for reactive oxygen species (ROS); i.e., our cellular biology interacts with the external environment to protect us against ROS. The composition of atmospheric oxygen reached its zenith at around 35% approximately 300 million years ago. By the late Paleozoic, it was 15%, and for the past 150 million years, it has leveled out at 21% (116). Biochemical evolution countered the oxygen threat by developing efficient aerobic catabolism (117). Despite this, the threat of a free radical attack still persists. A free radical is a highly reactive molecular species with an unpaired electron in its outer orbit. A reaction that involves a radical will generate another radical unless two radicals react together, which is actually unlikely because of low cellular concentrations of radicals and their extremely short half-life (nano-to picoseconds). As a result, free radical reactions form self-perpetuating chain reactions. It is worth noting that the major radicals that cause tissue damage are oxygen radicals. These are mainly the superoxide ($^{\bullet}O_2{}^-$), perhydroxyl ($^{\bullet}O_2H$), and hydroxyl ($^{\bullet}OH$) radicals. As I mention below in discussing senescence, anionic $^{\bullet}O_2{}^-$ is a particular problem, as it is constantly produced as part of mitochondrial respiration (Figure 5.1). It seems reasonable to view human antioxidant defences as an evolutionary adaptation to ROS. The mechanism for vitamin C quenching of ROS has been given earlier, but polyphenolic antioxidants like vitamin E work by delocalizing a single unpaired electron through a system of conjugated double bonds. The resultant radical is relatively stable and fairly unreactive. It persists long enough to be quenched and terminate the chain reaction of radical formation by interacting

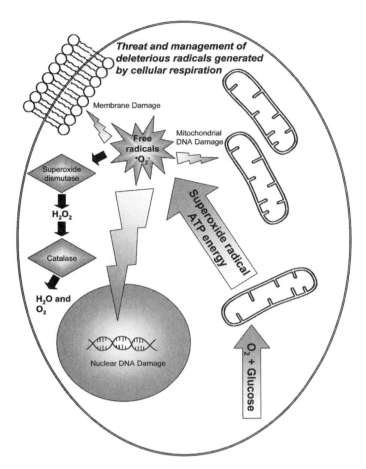

**Figure 5.1.** Scheme showing the built-in mechanism by which the cell deals with reactive oxygen species generated by cellular respiration. Although dietary antioxidants are a crucial defense mechanism against deleterious damage to DNA structure and membrane integrity, the superoxide dismutase system is considered to be the frontline built-in protection for the cell's delicate molecular organization.

with another "stable" radical. However, there is no doubt that the fallibility inherent in our antioxidant defense system is responsible for senescence and its associated morbidities. Benzie (117) contends that this shortfall in antioxidant potential stems from the fact that adaptive changes are selected for on the basis of reproductive benefit in relation to metabolic cost. As a consequence, the evolution of our endogenous antioxidant potential has not yet progressed beyond the "break-even" point of cost effectiveness. The obvious corollary is that the oxidant:antioxidant equilibrium always favors deleterious oxidation.

Early man dined on a banquet of plant-derived antioxidants. The photosynthetic process generates high levels of ROS within the chloroplast, as a consequence of which, plants have evolved elaborate quenching systems to neutralize these damaging species. To give an example, sites within plants that are prone to oxidative stress can have levels of vitamin C up to $1000\times$ that found in human plasma. Levels of vitamin C also increase due to wounding, growth, fruit maturation, and environmental stress (117). The tocopherols and tocotrienols and carotenoids are equally important, as are compounds that are not dietary essentials for our species such as the colorful anthocyanidins and other polyphenolic antioxidant molecules.

This raises some interesting questions. Given the obvious importance of antioxidant vitamins, why do we simply not manufacture these molecules rather than have them as dietary essentials? It seems likely that it is easier to forage for the abundant types of food rich in such molecules rather than synthesize them *de novo*. Consider: If dietary antioxidants were widely available, selection pressures would not act on metabolism to produce them endogenously. This may be true for many antioxidants such as vitamin E, but it is not the case for vitamin C.

Vitamin C is a puzzling nutrient, particularly in the context of human evolution. The enigma is as follows: Almost all species apart from humans and our primate relatives, guinea pigs, and birds manufacture vitamin C *de novo*. We cannot synthesize vitamin C because the gene encoding the terminal step in vitamin C biosynthesis, L-gulono-lactone oxidase, is inactive in humans, creating the dilemma of "what kind of evolutionary advantage is conferred by a mutation that prevents biosynthesis of such an important biomolecule?"

Scientists have tried to explain this evolutionary dilemma (118–123), which has been comprehensively reviewed by Benzie (117). It could shift the average population age down to enhance fertility, protect against hemolytic glucose-6-phosphate dehydrogenase deficiency in areas where malaria is endemic, accelerate evolution via increased exposure of DNA to ROS, and enhance the efficacy of our early immune response. These hypotheses are unlikely, however, and the best explanation probably resides in positive selection for an inactivation of the L-gulono-lactone oxidase gene, perhaps in a staged downregulation. This would fit into a paradigm of optimizing metabolic efficiency by using dietary sources of vitamin C, which exist in abundance. The metabolic cost of manufacturing vitamin C *de novo* might then, over the course of time, be diverted to a more pressing biochemical process. This argument is strengthened by the fact that noxious hydrogen peroxide is produced as part of vitamin C biosynthesis (124). The evolutionary loss of the *de novo* pathway means that the implementation of further antioxidant processes to remove this hydrogen peroxide were rendered redundant. It is interesting to note that loss of the *de novo* ascorbic acid pathway may have represented an evolutionary chiasma where uric acid supplants ascorbic acid as one of the body's main antioxidants (125,126). Water-soluble uric acid is a ubiquitous product of purine catabolism, which humans cannot metabolize on to allantoin like other organisms, because we do not possess the enzyme uricase. Care is required: Theories such as this need to be counterbalanced: ROS are a necessary part of important cellular mechanisms such as signal transduction pathways and redox-controlled transcription (127–130), so evolutionary selection may well have encouraged equilibrium in favor of a more pro-oxidant intracellular milieu, and this is why *de novo* ascorbic acid synthesis was dropped. However, in either scenario, it is fair to assume that reducing *de novo* derived intra- and extracellular ascorbic acid levels may have improved our biological fitness.

The importance of essential micronutrients is well described in this text, and it is emphasized by the various vitamin deficiency diseases. However, two vitamins that exemplify the notion that ascorbic acid may have evolved to become a vitamin, i.e., a dietary essential, is given by panthothenic acid and biotin—two vitamins that we take for granted because they are simply so abundant that deficiency is largely unknown except under extraordinary circumstances. Indeed, panthothenic acid means literally, "available everywhere." Clearly, mechanisms for the synthesis of such ubiquitous dietary molecules by man would be unnecessary and a waste of valuable cellular resources (as may be the case with vitamin C). Because all other essential vitamins are less abundant in our contemporary diet, deficiency states involving these important micronutrients are more easily attained than with panthothenic acid and biotin. However, our ancestral diet may well have been sufficiently rich in these molecules for evolution to act upon cellular metabolism in the ways I have described, and forge the metabolome we have today.

# Chapter 6

# Evolved Refinement of the Human Lifecycle Based on Nutritional Criteria

## 6.1 HUMAN BREAST MILK—AN EVOLVED FOOD

In the West, we tend to live in a world of instant gratification, a fairly synthetic world that is dominated by simple and instant solutions to problems: Broadband Internet can immediately address any question you throw at its search engines, a quick phone call and you can have a take-away meal delivered within 20 minutes, etc. It matters not that the information obtained from the Web may have little credibility, or that the take-away may be energy-rich–nutrient-poor junk. Such are the demands of our 24/7 lifestyles today that everyone of us has a need for immediate gratification, a process that is heavily modified by the influences of media advertising—*this food is better as a consequence of ..., this nutrient supplement is better because....* Clearly, as a species, we have adopted a different way of doing things to that of our ancestors, one that works in the short term, but that is far removed from the lifestyle that our bodies evolved to.

One of the most obvious nutritional distinctions between our ancestors and modern man is in the provision of breast milk versus formula for infant nutrition. Human breast milk is a perfect nutrient cocktail, biologically contrived to flawlessly meet the needs of the growing infant. Early man, like some of the few contemporary hunter-gatherer communities that still exist in our world (i.e., Kalahari !Kung), provided their infants with a continuous food supply; that is, nursing mothers carried their young in intimate proximity throughout their day's activities—often in a sling that permitted nursing on-demand. It has been suggested that this ancient practice that can be continued for up to 3 years might explain why modern human babies, which are weaned much earlier, like to be rocked when tearful. Furthermore,

*Molecular Nutrition and Genomics: Nutrition and the Ascent of Humankind*, by Mark Lucock
Copyright © 2007 John Wiley & Sons, Inc.

it has been suggested that being in constant bodily contact with their mothers who are able to read the early signs of distress and hunger, and having the convenience and proximity of an on-demand food source, obviates some of the behavioral traits exhibited by modern human infants. That is, they seldom cry, and they are less prone to colic. It has been suggested that colic may be a product of treating the infant of a species that is essentially a continuous feeder as if it were a spaced feeder (certainly the nutrient composition of breast milk is considered to be consistent with that of a continuous feeder). The adoption of our modern lifestyle has, in effect, turned the nursing mother from a provider of continuous breast milk into one that provides spaced feeding. The result of this is that the infant continues to thrive, albeit with an increase in the relatively minor physiologic response to more intermittent breast feeding—colic, tearfulness, etc.,—but the mother is provided with the opportunity of time to engage in other aspects of community life. Indeed, primates facilitate such a compromise for lactating mothers via elaborate social behavior such as the adoption of communal nursing. Clearly, although this train of thought regarding early infant nutrition seems valid, the conclusions are by their very nature speculative. However, the clear differences in the composition of breast and formula milks point to a less speculative conclusion that nature wins over nurture with respect to its "evolved for purpose" role and obvious health benefits.

The composition of breast milk can tell us a lot about a species and the environment in which it lives. Cold-water marine mammals have milk with a very high fat content; bats that have a low body mass to permit flight have milk that is low in water. The carbohydrate content of milk is high in primates due their need for rapid early brain development. Mammals that are born with a fully developed brain tend to have far less carbohydrate in the maternal milk. So what are the health advantages of human breast milk over formula?

- The nutrient composition of human breast milk is perfectly optimized for the infant via millions of years of evolution.
- Nutrient bioavailability has been optimized.
- Breast milk contains hormones, enzymes, and growth factors.
- Breast milk is a rich source of immune factors.
- Breast milk can induce the intestinal mucosal barrier and prevent disease.
- Breast fed individuals have higher cognitive development indices.

Although commercially prepared infant formula is an acceptable alternative to mother's milk, the above list and Figures 6.1 and 6.2 show that differences clearly do exist.

Colostrum, a viscous, transparent yellowish fluid is the initial form of human breast milk post-partum. It is higher in protein and lower in fat than mature milk. Colostrum is exceptionally rich in immune factors that protect the vulnerable neonate from viral and bacterial infections, giving their own immune systems time to develop. Human colostrum contains *Lactobacillus bifidus* factor that actively promotes the colonization of the neonatal gut by *Lactobacillus bifidus*, a protective bacterium that inhibits the growth of an enteropathogenic gut microflora. Infants fed on human breast milk have a gut microflora that is soon dominated by bifidobacteria. This can be contrasted with formula-fed infants whose gut microflora has many other enterobacterial species as well as bifidobacteria at one month postpartum; the gut ecology of a formula-fed infant is far more complex than that of a breast-fed infant. The metabolite profile of the intestinal microflora is in part determined by the bacterial composition of the gut, and there is now a general consensus that the character of the gut

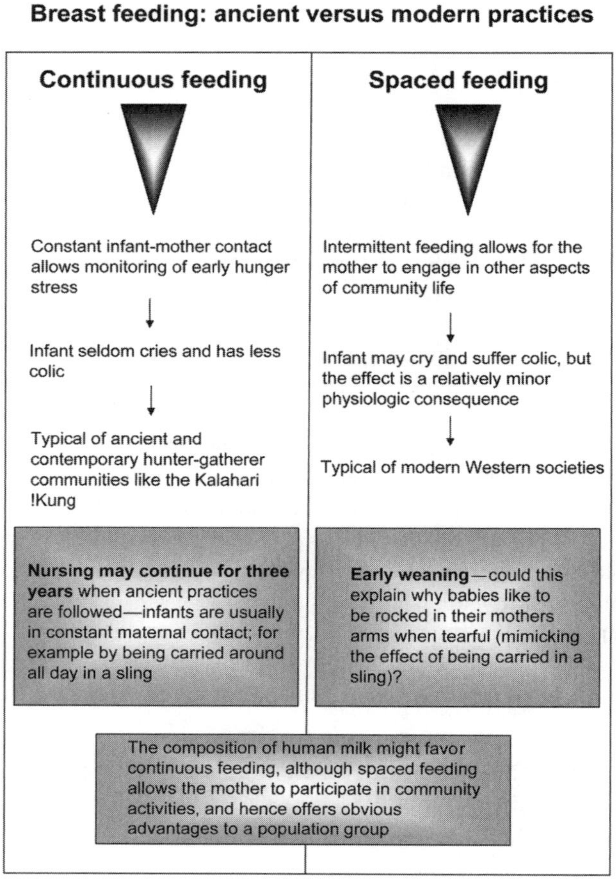

**Breast feeding: ancient versus modern practices**

| **Continuous feeding** | **Spaced feeding** |
| --- | --- |
| Constant infant-mother contact allows monitoring of early hunger stress | Intermittent feeding allows for the mother to engage in other aspects of community life |
| ↓ | ↓ |
| Infant seldom cries and has less colic | Infant may cry and suffer colic, but the effect is a relatively minor physiologic consequence |
| ↓ | ↓ |
| Typical of ancient and contemporary hunter-gatherer communities like the Kalahari !Kung | Typical of modern Western societies |
| **Nursing may continue for three years** when ancient practices are followed—infants are usually in constant maternal contact; for example by being carried around all day in a sling | **Early weaning**—could this explain why babies like to be rocked in their mothers arms when tearful (mimicking the effect of being carried in a sling)? |

The composition of human milk might favor continuous feeding, although spaced feeding allows the mother to participate in community activities, and hence offers obvious advantages to a population group

**Figure 6.1.** *The nature of breast feeding has changed over the millennia and differs between contemporary yet primitive cultures and mainstream Western societies. Figure 6.1 shows the salient differences in ancient versus modern practices of breast feeding.*

microflora affects pH, redox potential, and modulates gut maturation, integrity, competitive interactions with pathogens, and immune modulation.

Within six days, colostrum evolves into transitional milk, and within two weeks, the transformation to mature milk is complete. Where a mother's nutrient status is compromised, it is milk volume rather than quality that is diminished first. Figure 6.2 illustrates the biologically active molecules in human breast milk that aid neonatal development, and which, in some cases, set it apart from formula. Formula products tend to have a differing ratio of whey to casein. However, the more this ratio increases from that found in cow's milk, the closer it approaches that in human milk, and the smaller and more digestible is the curd formed in the stomach. The vitamin content of formula is often actually higher than that of human milk. The issue of using soymilk is dealt with later.

In summary, it seems that close, continuous, and prolonged nursing practices that evolved out of our early hunter-gatherer lifestyle (indeed, may be even before this), and that are still seen in sub-Saharan Africa in the Kalahari !Kung culture today, provide a more natural and harmonious vehicle for the provision of essential nutriture to the suckling infant. Although

**Some biologically active components in human breast milk that
aid neonatal development**

FATS

• The long-chain polyunsaturated fatty acid, docosahexaenoic acid, is concentrated in the retina and brain, and thus it is considered critical for cerebral development. Similarly, long-chain polyunsaturated fatty acids may be important in promoting antibacterial, antiviral, and antiprotozoan activity. Important forms include C12:0, C18:1, and C18:2.
• Formula products have recently become available that contain docosahexaenoic acid to mimic breast milk activity.
• The triacylglycerol content of breast milk is around 3.0–4.0 g/dL.

PROTEINS AND AMINO ACIDS

• Breast milk contains the immunoglobulins; secretory IgA, IgA, IgE, IgG, and IgM, which counter bacterial invasion of the gut and its mucosa. sIgA (50–100 mg/dL) is the predominant immunoprotein in human milk.
• Anti-staphylococccus factor inhibits the growth of potentially pathogenic *staphlococcal* infections.
• Bifidus factor promotes the growth of bifidobacteria that antagonize gut colonization by pathogens.
• Interferon in human milk acts as an antiviral agent by inhibiting viral replication.
• Lactoferrin binds iron and hence decreases the availability of iron for iron-requiring bacterial pathogens. This anti-infective therefore counters replication of pathogenic enterobacteria.
• Lactoperoxidase in breast milk is used to kill pathogenic *streptococci* and enteric bacterial species.
• Lysozyme is an anti-infective that kills bacteria by attacking the pathogen's cell wall.
• Lipase assists in fat digestion.
• Vitamin $B_{12}$ binding protein reduces the availability of this vitamin for bacterial cell division.
• Lactalbumin acts as a carrier of essential calcium irons.
• Casein is lower in human than cow's milk and is needed for carriage of Ca, P, Zn, Fe, and Cu ions.
• Human milk has more tyrosine, cystine, and taurine than cow's milk, perhaps due to neonatal inefficiency at synthesis of these amino acids.

CARBOHYDRATES

• Around 6-g lactose per 100-mL breast milk provides a major source of energy for the neonate. Infants with lactase deficiency can have lactose-free formula products made from corn syrup, sucrose, or modified tapioca starch as an alternative carbohydrate energy source.
• Polysaccharides can inhibit pathogenic bacterial attachment to the gut wall and hence colonization of the gastrointestinal tract.

CELLS

• Lymphocytes play an important role in synthesizing immune-proteins (i.e., sIgA).
• Macrophages synthesize lactoferrin and lysozyme. They perform phagocytosis.

**Figure 6.2.** *Some of the biologically active components that are found in human breast milk and that aid neonatal development. These include a range of important fatty acids and immune factors.*

modern practices are effective, they may have minor drawbacks associated with spaced feeding, less contact, and a greater reliance on synthetic milk products that lack, in particular, key immune factors (Figure 6.3).

## 6.2 CONFLICT BETWEEN PARENT AND OFFSPRING OVER NUTRIENT REQUIREMENTS

Parent–offspring conflict begins in the womb and is based on genetic asymmetry: Selection favors mothers that invest less time and energy than their infant's desire, and infants who demand more than their mothers are willing to provide. This process begins when

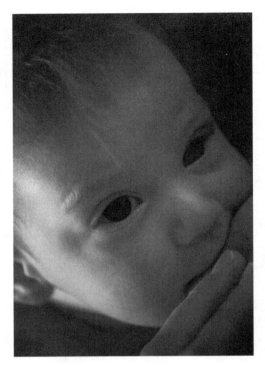

**Figure 6.3.** *Suckling infant. Human neonates probably evolved as continuous feeders, although modern practices tend to favor spaced feeding. This may account for the higher incidence of colic and tearfulness in Western infants compared with infants from contemporaneous hunter-gatherer communities that still adhere to continuous feeding practices.*

the embryo/fetus determines whether the pregnancy can be sustained, and subsequently it regulates the level and quality of nutrients that pass from the maternal to fetal circulation.

It is likely that mechanisms to elicit spontaneous abortion have evolved as adaptive responses. As sad as miscarriages are, they seem to exist as a quality control mechanism that ensures that most pregnancies carried to term are not associated with gross chromosomal abnormalities. More subtle genetic effects may also promote miscarriage: For example, two common SNPs of the MTHFR gene are C677T–MTHFR and A1298C–MTHFR. Most individuals will have no more than two mutant alleles shared among these SNPs within this single gene. Indeed, three mutant alleles are very rare and four unknown in research carried out by this author. It would seem that the protein cannot sustain its function if more than two mutant alleles are present in this MTHFR haplotype.

Maternal fitness at conception is likely to be important, because pregnancy is a costly investment; the expectant mother requires more food, and in ancestral humans, parturition was a major source of mortality. The cost of a pregnancy is greatest where genetic malformations in the embryo and/or poor maternal nutritional status halt translocation of nutrients to the embryo. Clearly, in either event, the biological cost of the pregnancy outweighs the benefits of having a child carrying a copy of the maternal genes. In such cases, natural selection promotes spontaneous abortion during the first trimester to conserve maternal energy reserves in favor of future pregnancies. The extent to which a mother eats for two is of interest. Mothers with elevated glucose produce larger, healthier offspring, but risk developing late-onset diabetes. The regulation of insulin as a mediator of glucose is the subject of a significant feto-maternal conflict: The fetus produces human placental lactogen to counter the effectiveness of the mother's insulin response. This is thought to be an attempt on the part of the fetus to raise blood sugar levels. The mother counters this by increasing the amount of insulin she produces. A similar feto-maternal conflict occurs for calcium. A flux of calcium from the maternal to fetal soluble pool, and on to the fetal skeleton is maintained at the expense of maternal skeletal calcium. It has been suggested that this evolutionary conflict arises because imprinting of renal GNAS (gene encoding G-protein $\alpha$-subunit) permits a marginal redistribution of calcium from fetus to mother, and it is associated with enhanced maternal fitness (131).

## 6.2.1  Imprinting and Allele Competition

Dietary folic acid, vitamins $B_{12}$, $B_2$, and $B_3$, are all likely to be important in the *de novo* genesis of methyl groups required for the regulated expression of DNA (see Figure 6.4). CpG-rich regions are found at the start of many genes. Undermethylation of these regulatory regions tends to promote transcription to RNA, whereas methylation tends to silence gene expression.

Imprinting is an important determinant of phenotype and results from embryonic identification of the parental origin for each allele, and the subsequent uniparental (monoallelic) expression of that gene (sometimes referred to as allelic exclusion). CpG methylation patterns are the language of imprinting, and when an active allele is lost, it leads to disease despite the presence of a normal allele that has been switched off by imprinting on the other chromosome. The best example of this is given by Angelman syndrome from a loss of maternal genetic material and Prader–Willi syndrome from a loss of paternal genetic material. What is fascinating about this is that you have different syndromes for the loss of the same gene with the same DNA sequence, but from alleles derived from different sexes. Individuals with Angelman syndrome are mentally retarded and suffer from uncontrolled laughter and rigid puppet-like gestures. This is in contrast to individuals suffering from Prader–Willi syndrome who have a milder mental retardation and tend toward extreme obesity.

The evolutionary force driving this is thought to be competition between genes from female and male parents (Figure 6.5). When male genes are switched on, it seems to offer an advantage to the embryo/fetus. For example, a larger placenta might offer advantages in the translocation of nutrients from the mother to the fetus. This is thought to modify behavior and promote sibling rivalry. The counterbalances for this are female genes that are activated to yield an equable balance of resources between offspring. Several human imprinted genes have been shown to be involved in fetal and placental growth, and imprinting defects can lead to embryonic and developmental defects, as well as to cancer.

Although the allele from one parent is selectively deactivated at an early stage of human development, the precise details of this process are still being elucidated. Given the importance of methyl groups and pyrimidines at a time of rapid cell growth and division, it seems that B-vitamin nutrients may be an important environmental factor in this exquisite mechanism of molecular-driven evolution.

Somewhere between 100 and 200 genes in the human genome are thought to be imprinted. The mechanism of CpG methylation and gene regulation probably emerged 150 million years ago in mammals. However, the reasons for the appearance and maintenance of this phenomenon through recent organic evolution remain controversial (133).

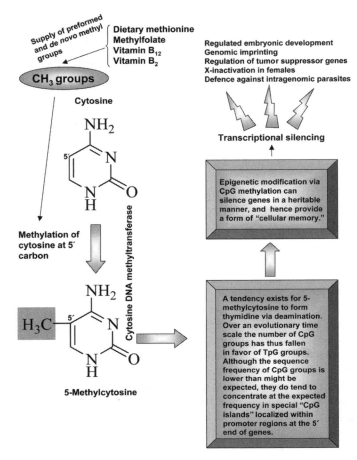

**Figure 6.4.** *Dietary factors play an important role in the provision of preformed and de novo methyl groups needed for maintaining DNA methylation patterns (CpG methylation). DNA methylation status provides a cellular memory and modulates gene transcription.*

## 6.2.2  The Thrifty Phenotype, a Model to Explain the Developmental Origins of Health and Adult Disease

Broadly speaking, dietary influences can modify phenotype over either a short or long time frame. A long evolutionary time course permits dietary/environmental selection pressures to act on the human genome in a heritable manner, and to select a range of possible thrifty traits, whereas one of the more immediate short-term effects thought to confer thriftiness is that which embodies the concept of the "developmental origins of health and adulthood disease," sometimes referred to as the "thrifty phenotype hypothesis" (see Figure 6.6).

It seems that poor fetal nutrition as a consequence of either restricted maternal dietary intake or perturbations in placental nutrient translocation may lead to adaptations in fetal metabolism that augment short-term survival. It is postulated that these adaptations in metabolism become permanent and lead to an altered physiological structure that creates a thrifty phenotype that affords a lifetime's advantage under marginal nutrient intake and status, but is at a clear disadvantage where nutrient intake becomes unrestricted in adulthood.

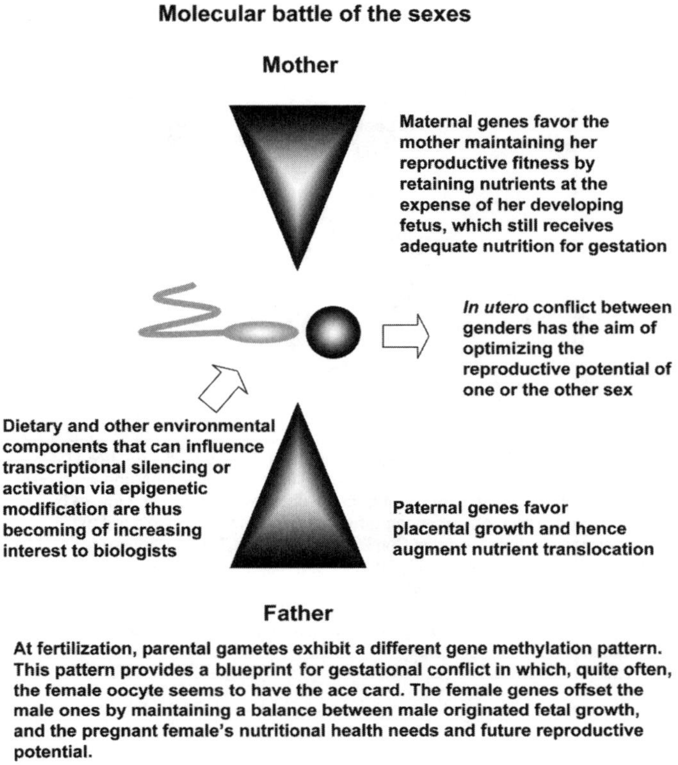

**Molecular battle of the sexes**

**Mother**

Maternal genes favor the mother maintaining her reproductive fitness by retaining nutrients at the expense of her developing fetus, which still receives adequate nutrition for gestation

*In utero* conflict between genders has the aim of optimizing the reproductive potential of one or the other sex

Dietary and other environmental components that can influence transcriptional silencing or activation via epigenetic modification are thus becoming of increasing interest to biologists

Paternal genes favor placental growth and hence augment nutrient translocation

**Father**

At fertilization, parental gametes exhibit a different gene methylation pattern. This pattern provides a blueprint for gestational conflict in which, quite often, the female oocyte seems to have the ace card. The female genes offset the male ones by maintaining a balance between male originated fetal growth, and the pregnant female's nutritional health needs and future reproductive potential.

**Figure 6.5.** *A molecular battle of the sexes begins at the earliest stages of the human lifecycle. This gender conflict proceeds during gestation, and likely optimizes the reproductive potential of one or the other sex.*

The thrifty phenotype hypothesis was initially developed to explain clinical associations between poor fetal and infant growth and the subsequent development of late onset (type 2) diabetes and the metabolic syndrome. The belief being that inadequate nutrition early in life yields permanent changes in glucose–insulin metabolism.

Although this work is of considerable interest, more recent work has also suggested that season of birth might even affect the early development of brain mechanisms that underpin eating behavior and weight. Although a fascinating area of enquiry, the idea that seasonal change in diet (i.e., vitamin intake) and sunlight exposure might affect early cerebral development and hence mood and psychopathology are not new, and have been in existence since the 1920s. Current research indicates that biological temporal rhythms such as exposure to daylight and hence melatonin production could impact on the developing fetus according to genotype in a manner that predicts weight gain and obesity. Robert Levitan et al. (132) have referred to this as the "seasonal thrifty phenotype hypothesis." In their paper (epub ahead of print at the time of writing), they show how the 7-repeat allele of the dopamine-4 receptor gene interacts with birth season to predict obesity in women with seasonal affective disorder.

The concept of a seasonal or other thrifty phenotype along with phenomena such as imprinting and allele competition are examples of where short-term environmental factors

## The thrifty phenotype model

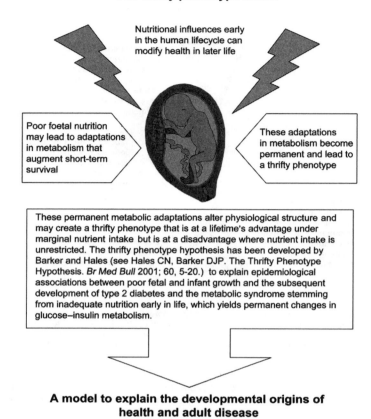

Nutritional influences early in the human lifecycle can modify health in later life

Poor foetal nutrition may lead to adaptations in metabolism that augment short-term survival

These adaptations in metabolism become permanent and lead to a thrifty phenotype

These permanent metabolic adaptations alter physiological structure and may create a thrifty phenotype that is at a lifetime's advantage under marginal nutrient intake but is at a disadvantage where nutrient intake is unrestricted. The thrifty phenotype hypothesis has been developed by Barker and Hales (see Hales CN, Barker DJP. The Thrifty Phenotype Hypothesis. *Br Med Bull* 2001; 60, 5–20.) to explain epidemiological associations between poor fetal and infant growth and the subsequent development of type 2 diabetes and the metabolic syndrome stemming from inadequate nutrition early in life, which yields permanent changes in glucose–insulin metabolism.

## A model to explain the developmental origins of health and adult disease

**Figure 6.6.** *The thrifty phenotype hypothesis describes how the nutritional environment of the embryo/fetus leads to an adaptive metabolic plasticity that affords short-term survival, but may, in the long-term, adversely influence adult health. This represents an important putative influence of nutrient availability that influences phenotype in the short term, as distinct from longer run in-effects due to more conventional evolutionary forces. Therefore, nutritional influences early in the human lifecycle likely modify health in later life using this paradigm to explain the developmental origins of adult health and disease.*

can potentially influence the long-term clinical phenotype in a manner that is clearly related to nutritional parameters.

## 6.3 NATURAL SELECTION FOR FORAGING EFFICIENCY

The hypotheses that relate to foraging efficiency are less relevant to contemporary Western societies than they were to our ancestral stock, although it has been applied to nomadic foragers that still exist in certain remote locations today. The theory of optimal foraging generates quantitative predictions that can be tested. The Aché are hunter-gatherers who, until the 1970s, lived a nomadic life in the forests of Paraguay. Studies have shown that their foraging behavior conforms to optimum foraging models, because they steer their resources to a higher rate of return in terms of calories expended per unit time than might be expected to occur on average (134). What is interesting is that two exceptions to optimal foraging theory were found in the Aché. First, males regularly ignored plant foods that would clearly increase their foraging efficiency over and above that achieved by seeking out fresh meat; and second, females had a tendency to ignore honey and meat, either of which would increase their foraging efficiency over that which would be achieved from their normal foraging target of plant foods. One explanation as to why men hunt more and gather less is the potential social pay-off in terms of improvements in their reproductive success. Indeed, reproductive and foraging success is correlated in male Aché, and the group benefits this provides include a degree of alloparenting, possibly as a trade off against extra food resources available to the whole group (134).

As today's environment offers us ready access to very high quality food with little energy expenditure involved in obtaining that food, we can only really learn about the evolution of control of food intake by studying extant populations such as the Aché, or by examining/extrapolating fossil evidence. Certainly an evolutionary perspective on how human fitness varies with food intake as an aggregate effect of its costs and benefits will help to formulate answers to these important questions (135). In maintaining a balanced perspective on the role of nutrition in human evolution, one needs to apply a degree of reductionism to explain molecular mechanisms that underpin any broad hypothesis. For instance, in the context above, the hypothalamic neuropeptides orexin-A and B regulate appetite control, but also increase EEG arousal, pain threshold, wakefulness, locomotor, and grooming activities in rats. Quite clearly, it would be a highly adaptive trait that allows the orexin system to be switched on in severe nutritional depletion. Predatory hunters that are hungry are driven to seek sustenance, but they are also more alert to environmental and competitive dangers. Mechanisms of this kind conspire and have evolved to provide effective foraging in humans, but they are obviously placed out of their appropriate context in modern society.

## 6.4 EVOLUTION OF SENESCENCE

Quite clearly, natural selection works less efficiently on traits that affect only the aged in society, because it will have a negligible influence on reproductive performance. Selection against a deleterious trait may be 30% less effective for a 50-year-old compared with a 20-year-old (134). A combination of two hypotheses best explains the evolution of aging: "*Antagonistic pleiotropy*" in which pleiotropic genes affording positive characteristics early in life and negative ones later in life favor selection of the aging process as does "*mutation accumulation*." In the latter case, aging results from the accumulation of mutations that affect only older individuals. That is, aging is not an adaptation, but a side effect of the fact that selection of traits that affect the old act as a fairly weak force (134).

The balance between free radicals generated largely from (1) the reoxidation of reduced flavins that occurs within mitochondria and as part of hepatic detoxification, (2) the macrophage respiratory burst, (3) formation of nitric oxide, and (4) nonenzymic formation; and protective mechanisms against radicals such as dietary antioxidants, protein binding and enzyme systems such as SOD, and glutathione peroxidase do much to regulate the aging process. DNA repair mechanisms are also crucial: *DNA Polymerase 1* catalyses template-directed synthesis of DNA with its exonuclease activity filling in single-strand gaps and hydrolyzing mismatch base pairs.

*Direct DNA repair* is also important, although it does not remove aberrant bases but corrects the damage—for example, alkyltransferase reverses alkylation of the O-6 position of guanine, whereas photolyases can reverse UV-induced pyrimidine dimers. *Excision repair* is a mechanism by which mutation-induced dimensional distortion of the DNA double helix is recognized. The outcome is that excinuclease cuts the DNA backbone, removing a tiny oligonucleotide section containing the lesion, and repairs the strand with DNA polymerase and DNA ligase. Many types of *glycosylase* such as uracil glycosylase specifically cleave uracil and are often related to problems with folate availability, for example, where uracil has been misincorporated into DNA instead of thymine when folate status is inadequate. Others remove hypoxanthine, alkylated bases, or pyrimidine dimers. The action of glycosylases must be repaired by endonucleases. *Mismatch repair* occurs after replication; mismatched base pairs are removed from the newly synthesized strand because the template DNA is methylated and can be discriminated from the parent strand. Folate status has recently been linked to this mechanism as a way of regulating programmed cell death (apoptosis) (40).

A full account of aging is beyond the scope of this book, although many experts believe that chromosomal telomere length and mitochondrial DNA damage provide two of the best indices of the aging process. The role of antioxidants on ameliorating the aging process due to nuclear -, mitochondrial DNA, and membrane damage should never be underestimated; overexpression of a single gene, SOD1, in a single cell type, the motor neuron, extends the normal fruit fly lifespan by up to 40% and rescues the lifespan of short-lived SOD null mutant flies. Elevated resistance to oxidative stress suggests that the lifespan extension observed in these flies is due to enhanced reactive oxygen metabolism (136).

Clearly, the various aging processes are many fold. However, if aging is due to antagonistic pleiotropy, the various aging phenomena should exist in synchrony (134). That is, selection will favor postponement of the expression of genes that augment one aspect of the aging process so that they synchronize with other age-causing cellular processes. Alternatively, it might favor earlier onset of the other cellular aging factors; in either event, it would lead to the simultaneous expression of aging phenomena.

Thus, if aging does arise via antagonistic pleiotropy, eradicating one or a few of the aging mechanisms may not lead to an indefinitely long lifespan. In contrast, if mutation accumulation is responsible for regulating longevity, the random process of mutations arising would not be synchronized to the various mutation-related causes of aging. In this case, eradicating the effects of these mutations may substantially extend lifespan (134).

These theories can help explain the evolution of senescence, but they do not account for the premature end to the female menstrual cycle at around 50 years of age, particularly given a women's life expectancy of 70+ years. It has been suggested that the seemingly odd process of menstruation evolved to permit the most energy-efficient mechanism of maintaining the uterus in a state of preparedness for pregnancy. To sustain the postovulation luteal phase, women consume considerably more calories than they do during the preovulatory follicular phase of their monthly cycle. Thus, from a nutritional perspective, it is energetically far less expensive to cycle receptiveness to pregnancy, than to sustain a state of constant receptiveness (137).

The onset of menopause is thought to be tied in to the level of nutrition experienced by women and varies among societies. It has been suggested that menopause may simply be an artifact of the very recent extension of the human lifecycle, although it may have evolved because postmenopausal women could play a more useful role in the care of their children and grandchildren. That is, they direct their resources to existing offspring rather than produce further children themselves. This ensures they live long enough to see their offspring through to independence, while permitting extra time in foraging activities that benefit the population group as a whole (138). This theory remains to be proven, and to date we cannot satisfactorily answer why women cease reproductive status so long before the end of their natural lifespan. To put it more effectively, why has a female reproductive system evolved for a 50-year life, whereas the major organs have evolved to last considerably longer? Blurton Jones et al. (139) explore whether postreproductive life is a phenotypic outcome of modern conditions. They conclude that the senescent phase of the postreproductive lifespan does indeed require some explanation. Caspari has gone further and suggests that patterns of hominid dental wear indicate a dramatic increase in longevity during the Early Upper Paleolithic, and that this is partially responsible for population expansions and cultural innovations associated with modernity (140).

# Chapter 7

# The Evolution of Human Disease

## 7.1 THE CONFLICT BETWEEN AGRICULTURE AND ANCESTRAL GENES

This section examines how an increase in brain size has led to our meteoric success as a species, but in the process, it has led to a modern lifestyle that is not compatible with our ancestral genes. Human genetic change does occur, but it is slow. Before examining this issue in depth, it is worth mentioning what I believe is one of the most interesting examples of molecular evolution illustrative of a positive selection pressure in mammalian nutrition. It does not involve humans, but it relates to another primate, the colobine monkey. Foregut evolution by placental mammals has arisen on two independent occasions: once in colobine monkeys and once in ruminants such as cows. In both scenarios, lysozyme is secreted into the stomach to aid in the degradation of bacterial cell walls. Despite the phylogenetic disparity between these species, their lysozyme has evolved independently as a series of seven parallel or convergent amino acid substitutions in the cow and monkey lineages (141). At a functional level, their lysozyme has evolved to work best at a low gastric pH value and is less able to function at the pH optima of human lysozyme. This example of how genes do invariably adapt is an elegant example of parallel adaptation to similar selective agents. Hopefully, humans will be around long enough for our nutrition-related genes to adapt to our intellect, and its overriding ability to permit our species to shape the environment to its requirements rather than the other way around as with all other creatures. Sadly, one could argue that this may be a philosophical impossibility.

Paleolithic man had genes well adapted to a lifestyle that was sustained on marine food, fruit, roots, legumes, green leaves, nuts, raw honey, and meat. This food was mostly uncooked and consumed almost immediately. What is clear is that neither grain nor dairy foods were consumed. This translates into a diet that probably contained two or three times the fiber, micronutrients, and phytochemical antioxidant content of a modern human diet

(142,143). The role of ancient, complex homeostatic mechanisms that our "stone age" genes confer is now partially redundant because these ancient genes are less effective in the context of modern nutritional and lifestyle practices. The human genome is a temporal mosaic: brain dimensions, developmental processes, speech, etc. have evolved very recently. By contrast, most human genes are even older than our genus itself. It is thought that any recent evolutionary pressure on our genome has not, by itself, impacted on the various chronic degenerative diseases that plague modern society; rather that it is our modern diet that differs so much from that which sustained our ancestors that is implicated in coronary heart disease and other degenerative conditions (144,145).

The root of much of our chronic adulthood disease is born out of a revolution that occurred 10,000 years ago in the Fertile Crescent that represents today's Middle East (Figure 7.1). The domestication and subsequent cultivation of wild strains of wheat growing in this region were able to sustain Neolithic tribes for the entire year on the harvested stored grain. This dependable food supply, along with the domestication of wild animals, offered many obvious advantages. Additionally, seasonal migrations to seek out food were no longer necessary, and static populations developed as the quaternary ice shield retreated. With this came culture, population growth, and the nascent origins of today's sophisticated social urban developments. As transportation mechanisms were primitive, food could not be moved any great distance, limiting community size. This fact not withstanding, cities of 50,000 developed quite quickly. European data are the most comprehensive and show that the benefits of an agriculturalist society led to the expansion of domesticated livestock and cultivated crops out from the Fertile Crescent of Southern Anatolia, Israel, Syria, Northern Iraq, and Western Iran around 9500 years ago. The spread was slow—around 1 km/year as the flow of agriculturalist genes diffused out from the Fertile Crescent. The dominant agriculturalists exhibit a partial admixture with isolated groupings of hunter-gatherers, which became absorbed, and show a concentric cline of genes emanating out from the Middle East consistent with a demic expansion of agriculture (*demic—of people rather than culture*) (146,147).

With the obvious benefits of agriculture came problems. A comparison of North American Indian physiognomy showed that genetically similar tribes that obtained their nutriture from either grain based agronomy or hunter-gatherer foraging differed. Agriculturalist Hardin villagers in the Ohio River Valley during AD 1500–1675 showed signs of chronic malnutrition, dental caries, and short stature, whereas hunter-gatherers that lived in the same area and climatic conditions 4500 years earlier were well nourished, had non-carious teeth and taller stature. This nutritional physiognomic pattern is mirrored today in parts of Africa (148,149).

With the Industrial Revolution came a sea change in nutriture for the masses. Inexpensive sources of white flour and white sugar became widely available. This led to a reduction in intake of micronutrients, fiber, and other useful phytochemicals. This calorie-rich, nutrient-poor diet led to the occurrence of so-called saccharine diseases during the twentieth century (Figure 7.2). Conditions such as diverticular disease, colorectal cancer, caries, diabetes, obesity, hypertension, and occlusive vascular disease are rare in primitive societies (149,150). To provide an example of the importance of one group of vitamins in the changing etiology of heart disease, one only has to consider three B-vitamins. In Paleolithic times, intake of folate, vitamins $B_6$ and $B_{12}$, have been calculated as around 350, 3500 and 15 $\mu$ per day—all significantly higher than in the United States and Europe at the end of the twentieth century. Refined wheat, sugar, and a highly processed diet during most of the twentieth century led to deficiencies in these three vitamins and a concomitant increase in blood homocysteine

**Transition of modern man from a hunter-gatherer to an agriculturalist and inhabitant of permanent settlements**

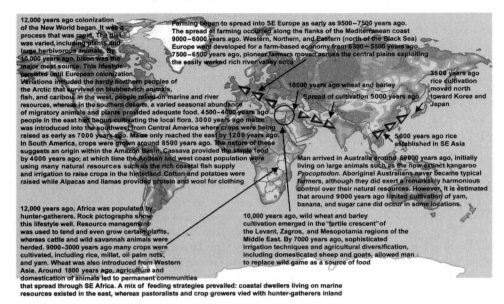

**Figure 7.1.** *The transition of modern man from a hunter-gatherer to an agriculturalist and inhabitant of permanent settlements spread across the globe. One of the most significant developments occurred 10,000 years ago in the "fertile crescent" of the Middle East where wild wheat and barley were first cultivated.*

(149) (see Figures 2.8 and 2.9). Given the significant role of homocysteine in heart disease, arteriosclerosis, and embryotoxicity, one can immediately see the discordance between a Western refined diet and our ancient genes.

The ratio of pre-agricultural $\omega$-6:$\omega$-3 fatty acids was around 1:1. This compares with 15:1 in today's Western culture. Although cholesterol was similar then and now, carbohydrates in Paleolithic times originated from fruit and vegetables, and not dairy products, cereals, and refined sucrose as today. The ancestral diet will also have been lower in sodium and higher in soluble and insoluble fiber and phytochemicals.

These differences in diet are significant: $\omega$-6:$\omega$-3 fatty acids today impact upon heart disease; fruits, vegetables, and phytochemicals are cancer preventative; and the ancient diet had the optimum contribution of fat to dietary energy (143).

## 7.1.1 Homocysteine and Modern Society

According to McCully (149,151), widespread deficiencies of vitamins $B_6$, folic acid, and vitamin $B_{12}$ arose because of consumption of refined wheat flour, sugar, and processed foods. Associated with this was an increase in blood homocysteine level that had serious consequences, leading to widespread arteriosclerosis and coronary heart disease. Recent population studies have shown that elevated homocysteine is indeed a potent risk factor for

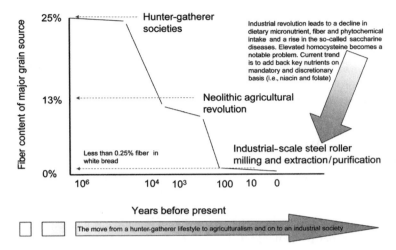

**Figure 7.2.** *Figure shows fiber consumption by humans as an indicator of the changing dietary trends of modern man—that is, over the past 1,000,000 years. Clearly, our dietary fiber content has steadily fallen since man became an agriculturalist, and particularly so since the mechanization procedures that were first associated with the industrial revolution.*

vascular disease and that deficiency of these critical B vitamins is common in populations at risk.

The homocysteine theory of arteriosclerosis is now well established. Indeed, a major decline in mortality from heart attacks in the United States in the last half-century is attributable to increased amounts of folic acid and vitamin $B_6$ as a consequence of voluntary fortification of grains and cereals. From this, it is therefore evident that a deficiency in these micronutrients arises when wheat and other foodstuffs are milled and processed into white flour, sugar, white rice, canned foods, and other highly processed food products (149,151).

The discovery that elevated homocysteine leads to occlusive vascular disease stems from important early work: An increase in both plasma and urinary homocysteine levels results from several inherited and nutritional diseases that affect homocysteine remethylation and transsulphuration (see Figure 2.8 and 2.9). Serum and urinary homocysteine levels in normal subjects are in the same low $\mu$mol/L range. Plasma homocysteine exists in sulphydryl and mixed disulphide form. Homocystinuria, as an inborn error of metabolism, was first described by Carson and Neill (152). Harvey Mudd et al. later showed a deficiency of cystathionine ß-synthase in liver biopsies taken from homocystinuric individuals (153). Other rare enzyme deficiencies leading to elevated homocysteine were subsequently elucidated. Homozygotes for this cystathionine ß-synthase defect experience mental retardation, thromboembolism, and premature arteriosclerosis, which present at any age (154). These findings were therefore an important clue to this thiol's potential vasculotoxicity.

Animal and human research work clearly link plasma homocysteine level with vascular disease; sustained homocysteine treatment in primates results in changes that mimic those observed in early human arteriosclerosis (155). Clinical research studies now support the experimental animal data, and they are consistent in their findings, which indicate patients with occlusive vascular disease have higher blood homocysteine than individuals with no disease. Despite this, most vascular patients have values within what had at one time been considered to be the normal range (156,157). In other words, levels do not need to rise too high before pathology ensues.

An extremely profound reciprocal linear relationship exists between blood homocysteine and blood B vitamins (particularly folate), and before the implementation of mandatory fortification of grain with folate in the United States, it had been calculated that 9% of male and 54% of female coronary artery deaths in that country (around 50,000 deaths/year) could be prevented by mandatory fortification of grain products with the synthetic pteroylmonoglutamic acid form of folic acid (158).

A few studies failed to find an association between plasma homocysteine and occlusive vascular disease (159,160); however, sufficient evidence now exists to support such an association (161–164). Even modest increases in plasma homocysteine have a significant pathological effect on vascular endothelium. However, although the best-documented effects of homocysteine toxicity are linked to arteriosclerosis, research has now shown homocysteine to exhibit a multitude of deleterious effects that are particularly important in brain, embryonic, as well as vascular tissue. These include not just arteriosclerosis and hypertension via oxidative challenge, but a damaging effect of homocysteine on connective tissue and procoagulant activity via several routes. Homocysteine is also considered embryotoxic and neurotoxic. Figure 7.3 shows the mechanisms involved in all these deleterious actions.

Further interest exists in homocysteine because of its association with a gene that encodes an important folate-dependent allosteric enzyme (5,10MTHFR) that may link folate to occlusive vascular disease via regulation of plasma homocysteine levels. This has been dealt with earlier, but it is worth mentioning again in a clearer vascular context: A common mutation of the gene coding for this enzyme (C677T-MTHFR) affects approximately 15% of people in its homozygous recessive form and is associated with elevated plasma homocysteine. It is also associated with a tiered reduction in 5,10MTHFR activity between genotypes (165), possibly indicating incomplete dominance at the biochemical level. Guenther et al. showed that folate coenzymes stabilize the variant protein expressed by C677T-MTHFR by preventing the polymorphic enzyme from relinquishing its flavin cofactor (43). Their model supports the treatment of hyperhomocysteinemia with folate, and it provides an elegant example of a nutrient–gene interrelationship, which may have profound health implications.

Although the modern Western diet may be far from perfect, at least discretionary and mandatory use of micronutrients is now beginning to alleviate hyperhomocysteinemia, although their use remains controversial. One can argue that achieving this kind of nutritional "norm" may well shift the genetic equilibrium toward evolutionary stasis. However, it is even more interesting to consider the opposite scenario. After the Second World War, a shortage of food led to famine. There was an increase in amenorrhea (loss of periods), presumably as a protective mechanism against a potential compromise in fetal nutrition were conception to occur. This has been taken to imply a lack of preparedness of these malnourished post-war women for pregnancy. It has been estimated that in the Netherlands, half of all women stopped menstruating. However, fertility was least affected in rural areas where fresh food was easier to find. The effect of this famine led to an increase in spontaneous abortions (miscarriages), stillbirths, congenital malformations, and neonatal mortality. One can postulate that homocysteine elevations may have played some role in this phenomenon, and that if this were not a transient effect, that this knife edge environmental pressure

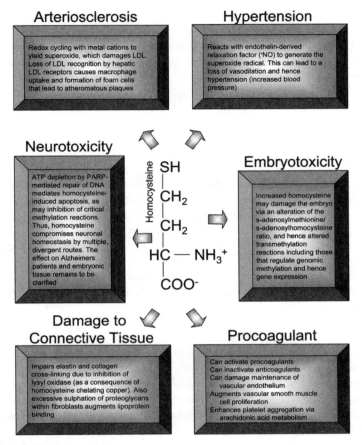

**Figure 7.3.** *Scheme showing the various mechanisms involved in the deleterious actions of homocysteine upon cellular processes.*

would have been likely to shift the equilibrium away from evolutionary stasis, perhaps with genes such as C677T-MTHFR having their homozygous recessive genotype removed from the population, with other advantageous alleles increasing to provide survival advantage. Within the human genome, around 40% of amino acid substitutions that occur in functional proteins are the result of positive selection.

Although the post-war years led to a decline in birth weight and length, these indices returned to normal by 1948.

## 7.2 OBESITY: A CHRONIC PLAGUE OF OUR AFFLUENT SOCIETIES

The plague of obesity and its comorbidities is well known in the West. However, it is also now becoming far more prevalent in the developing world. Since the turn of the century, and particularly since the end of World War II, obesity has emerged as a serious problem.

The problem began to surface when our diet changed from one rich in carbohydrates with only modest fat to one that is dominated by meat and dairy products rich in fats.

Being overweight means you are more likely to suffer premature death. The comorbidities of obesity include cardiovascular disease, dyslipidemia, gallbladder problems, hyperinsulinemia, hypertension, glucose intolerance, osteoarthritis, impaired fertility, sleep apnea, a variety of cancers, and non-insulin-dependent diabetes mellitus. By contrast, optimum life expectancy is met with a body mass index (BMI; weight/height$^2$) of 20–25. A BMI of 25–30 is consistent with being overweight, whereas a BMI of 30–40 would be considered obese. At this level of BMI, an obese individual is 20% to 60% heavier than they should be. To place this in context, one third of adults in the United States are considered to be clinically obese (166).

The consequence of industrialization and the information age have led to a rise in levels of urbanization and a far more sedentary workforce. Couple this decline in energy expenditure with unfettered access to calorie-rich foods, and you have a recipe for what has been termed as the "obesogenic" environment (167). What this refers to is a scenario in which obesity becomes a collective adaptation to the pathological environmental pressure to eat too much and exercise too little (168).

Susceptible members of Western societies who suffer from obesity within an obesogenic environment may have acquired this phenotype from their thrifty alleles. As outlined earlier, thrifty genes that predispose to obesity and its comorbidities in later life may actually have a selective advantage at an earlier phase of the human lifecycle within populations whose nutritional intake is precarious and/or erratic (169). Contemporary populations in which these thrifty genes are common include Pima Indians and Pacific Islanders (170). Also, environment and lifestyle fail to explain the higher rates of obesity in African- and Hispanic-Americans compared with Caucasians (171). Bell et al. provide a comprehensive review of the genetics of human obesity, and complex polygenic obesity (common obesity) that is caused by many different genes as well as environmental factors in a recent *Nature Genetics* Reviews article (168).

A small selection of the proteins encoded by genes (in brackets) that are associated with an obese phenotype include adipocyte C1Q and collagen domain containing adiponectin (ACDC); a variety of adrenergic receptor proteins (ADRA2A, ADRA2B, ADRB1, ADRB2, ADRB3); leptin receptor (LEPR); glucocorticoid receptor (NR3C1); peroxisome proliferative activated receptor-$\gamma$ (PPARG); and uncoupling proteins 1, 2, and 3 (UCP1, -2, and -3) (168).

## 7.3 PRION PROTEIN LOCUS AND HUMAN EVOLUTION: THE LINK BETWEEN VARIANT CREUTZFELD-JAKOB DISEASE AND CANNIBALISM

A fascinating idea has been put forward that our genes may actually contain a legacy of our cannibalistic past, and that this may impact on the expression of new variant Creutzfeld–Jakob Disease (vCJD) (172,173).

Prion proteins (PrP) are small glycoproteins dominated by three alpha helices normally found at the cell surface, within the plasma membrane. PrPC (C for cellular) is a normal body protein that has changed its three-dimensional configuration into one with a secondary structure dominated by a beta sheet conformation (PrPSc for scrapie). It is encoded by a gene designated (in humans) PRNP, which is located on chromosome 20. When PrPSc comes into contact with PrPC, it converts the PrPC into more of the abnormal PrPSc form.

Aggregates of these molecules then lead to cellular damage, although it is not clear whether these aggregates are themselves causal for, or simply a side effect of, the underlying disease process. In the United Kingdom, human vCJD appeared a few years after the devastating epidemic of Mad Cow Disease (bovine spongiform encephalitis BSE) swept through the country's cattle herds. The cattle and human prion protein gene, designated PRNP, differ at 30 codons within the gene. However, despite this, it would seem that patients with vCJD had acquired the disease from consuming beef products contaminated with the cattle prion.

The PRNP genotype of individuals with vCJD was examined. A genetic polymorphism that encodes either methionine or valine at codon 129 (M129V) was discovered. Quite remarkably, all patients with vCJD were homozygous for this "susceptibility" polymorphism and had a methionine at position 129 of the polypeptide.

From an evolutionary standpoint, however, it is most interesting to examine this SNP in the Fore linguistic tribe of Papua New Guinea. This population suffered from an acquired prion disease known as "kuru". Kuru was transmitted during endocannibalistic mortuary feasts where diseased relatives were consumed. This ritualistic feeding pattern led to the conversion of the normal PrPC prion into the abnormal PrPSc form of the protein and promoted spread of the spongiform encephalopathy that the Fore tribe knows as kuru. What is most interesting is that the older survivors of the kuru epidemic, who were participants at many mortuary feasts, are, by contrast to younger Fore, predominantly PRNP 129 heterozygotes.

These findings indicate that there is a distinct heterozygote advantage created by habitual cannibalistic rituals. Since the practice of cannibalism and the recycling of prions in the Fore population was halted, kuru has disappeared. Clearly, natural selection has increased the frequency of this protective genotype within populations that are exposed to prion disease, and in a sense, cannibalistic genes are therefore a (selectable) part of humankind's genetic makeup.

# Chapter 8

# *Contemporary Dietary Patterns that Work: The Mediterranean Diet*

There is little doubt that at a broad level, today's consumers are far more aware of the important relationship between diet and disease than ever before. It is popular knowledge that, for example, "the Mediterranean diet" is beneficial, whereas a diet of "pie and chips washed down with a pint of beer" is not. What is it about the Mediterranean diet, for example, that affords protection against cardiovascular disease and cancer (174–176)? Much research today is focused on specific food items of this traditional dietary pattern: grains: vegetables, fruit, and olive oil. The molecular components within these foods that are of greatest interest are most probably polyphenolic molecules, vitamins, oleic acid, and fiber.

## 8.1 TOMATOES

A brief resume of the functional food potential of these various "Mediterranean" biomolecules reveals obvious benefits. Tomatoes are rich in many useful nutrients, but of greatest interest in recent years is the almost unique occurrence in tomatoes of the non-provitamin A carotenoid, lycopene. Lycopene is a potent antioxidant that exhibits a strong inverse relationship with cancers of the prostate gland, lung, and stomach (177). It may be of some comfort to those who have a pizza-and-baked-beans-rich diet that processed tomato products are also a good source of lycopene. Tomatoes also contain other carotenoids such as $\beta$-carotene, lutein, and zeaxanthein. A diet high in lutein may reduce age-related macular degeneration. In humans, the pigment lutein is concentrated in the macula of the eye (part of the retina where the sharpest vision is rendered). Lutein works by neutralizing free radicals. What is interesting are the conflicting reports of the health benefits of carotenoids

*Molecular Nutrition and Genomics: Nutrition and the Ascent of Humankind*, by Mark Lucock
Copyright © 2007 John Wiley & Sons, Inc.

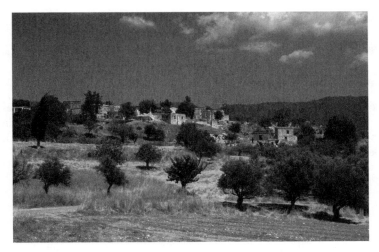

**Figure 8.1.** *Olive trees growing in the Mediterranean; olives represent part of a protective Mediterranean diet. The health benefits of olive oil are thought to stem from the monounsaturated fat, oleic acid, but they also contain other beneficial compounds like hydroxytyrosol and oleuropein, both polyphenolic antioxidants.*

(178–180). It seems that pro-oxidant and cancer promoting properties sometimes attributed to $\beta$-carotene supplements are not documented from studies on natural food sources of this phytoprotectant such as tomatoes (181). As the world moves toward overreliance on supplements and mandatory fortification for maintaining health, it is important to draw attention to the possibility that the health benefits of such foods as tomatoes are almost certainly not limited to its $\beta$-carotene content alone (182). It's far more likely that a blend of phytoprotectants interact in a synergistic manner to counter deleterious cellular challenges that precipitate chronic adulthood disease.

## 8.2 OLIVE OIL

Olive oil is the dominant source of fat in the typical Mediterranean diet (Figure 8.1). The health benefits of olive oil are thought to stem from the monounsaturated fat, oleic acid (18:1n-9). However, olives are also rich sources of polyphenols such as hydroxytyrosol and oleuropein, which are potent scavengers of ROS implicated in vascular disease and cancer. These molecules also modulate enzyme systems involved in coagulation and are thus potentially protective against both atherogenic and thrombogenic vascular disease (181).

## 8.3 RED WINE

One of the best-known aspects of the Mediterranean diet is the potentially protective role that moderate consumption of red wine confers. In the late 1970s it was noted that avid drinkers of red wine in France had less heart disease than other Western populations, even though they consumed more saturated fat in their diet. This became known as the "French Paradox". We now recognize that the presence of high concentrations of antioxidant polyphenolic bioflavonoids in red grape skins can help prevent vascular disease.

## 8.4 BIOFLAVONOIDS

There are many useful types of bioflavonoid in the typical Mediterranean diet (Figure 8.2).

### 8.4.1 Flavonols

The Mediterranean diet provides a variety of flavonols found in fruit, vegetables, and red wine, with onion being a very good source for this class of bioflavonoid, which include the bioactive molecules—quercetin, myricetin, and isohamnetin among its ranks. Quercetin-3-glucuronide, for example, can suppress phospholipid peroxidation.

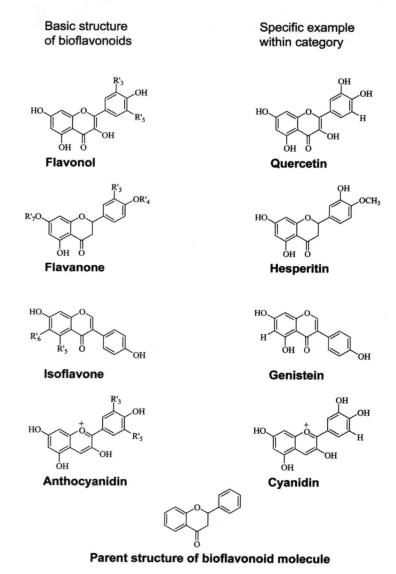

**Figure 8.2.** *Basic structures of the bioflavonoids common in the Mediterranean diet, including specific examples within each category.*

### 8.4.2  Flavanones

Flavanones are the predominant bioflavonoids found in citrus fruits like limes, lemons, grapefruits, and oranges. The citrus fruit flavanone compounds of most interest include hesperidin, nairirutin, naringin, eriocitrin, didymin, and poncirin. Citrus fruit flavanones have both anti-inflamatory and anti-cancer properties.

### 8.4.3  Proanthocyanins

One of the major groups of bioflavonoid consumed in the West are proanthocyanidins. Apples and grape seed extract are rich sources, as are fruits and berries in general. Proanthocyanidins decrease the susceptibility of LDL to oxidation and inhibit platelet function (183). The bioactive proanthocyanidins found in grape seeds induce apoptosis in human prostate cancer (184), with a cytotoxic influence on MCF-7 breast cancer cells, A-427 lung cancer cells, and gastric adenocarcinoma cells (185). Interestingly, they also beneficially enhance the metabolic capacity of normal cells. These molecules may also bind cholesterol and prevent its intestinal uptake. One of the best-known effects of proanthocyanidins is to inhibit the adhesion of pathogenic bacteria to the uroepithelial cells. Cranberry juice is best known for this "functional food" effect.

### 8.4.4  Anthocyanins

Anthocyanins are colorful and potent antioxidant bioflavonoids. Cyanidin is the most abundant anthocyanin and is found in 90% of all fruit, with the richest sources being the most strongly colored fruits—deep purple or black berries.

### 8.4.5  Isoflavones

The isoflavones are largely found in legumes with soybeans being the best-known source. These bioflavonoids are phytoestrogens, which have been discussed earlier, and are dealt with in much greater depth in the following section.

### 8.5  FISH

The intake of fish and fish oil products readily increases the body's eicosapentanoic acid (EPA) and docosahexaenoic acid (DHA) levels, including within the all important breast milk compartment. DHA is likely to be an important component of human breast milk because it is concentrated in the retina of the eye and the brain where it is crucial for the functional competency of embedded proteins (i.e., rhodopsin in the eye and postsynaptic proteins in the brain) (186). Its role in visual function and cognitive development is currently the subject of active research, particularly in respect of its "functional food" role in infant milk formula.

In the West, our current intake of DHA and EPA is of concern. Over the past century, our diet has changed dramatically. Most notably we have increased our intake of saturated fats, *trans*-fatty acids, and linoleic acid (LLA). This has been at the expense of a reduced intake of the n-3 fatty acids, which includes $\alpha$-linolenic acid (ALA) and a range of n-3 long-chain polyunsaturated fatty acids, particularly DHA and EPA (187).

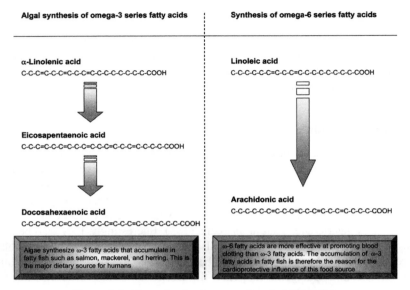

**Figure 8.3.** Biosynthesis of omega −3 and −6 fatty acids.

From a perspective that looks at the evolution of human pathology, neither LLA, nor ALA, can be synthesized in the body. They are therefore essential components of our diet. Both of these latter compounds undergo chain elongation, desaturation, and chain shortening to form their respective long-chain polyunsaturated fatty acid metabolites.

The Mediterranean diet is known for its marine component and is therefore replete in n-3 DHA and EPA. However, the most important n-6 long-chain polyunsaturated fatty acid is arachidonic acid (AA). This is also concentrated in the retina and brain, but it is mostly derived from dietary meat.

Both EPA and AA are precursors of transitory eicosanoids. These regulatory hormones play a key role in the inflammatory process, clotting, and blood pressure regulation (186). Figure 8.3 shows how DHA is synthesized within algae and accumulates in fatty fish (herring, mackerel, etc.), and how AA is synthesized from LLA. It is interesting to compare patterns of saturation: The Inuit have a traditional diet of extremely fatty foods rich in n-3 polyunsaturated fatty acids; yet they also have a low incidence of vascular disease. Eicosanoids derived from n-3 fatty acids are less effective at promoting blood clotting than n-6 fatty acids, and this may, at least in part, account for this population's resistance to vascular disease.

Polyunsaturated fatty acids and long-chain metabolites of LLA and ALA are also garnering interest for a nutrient–gene interaction in which they modulate transcription factors that help regulate metabolic processes such as cholesterol homeostasis and inflammation. They achieve this by interacting with the PPAR (peroxisome proliferator activated receptor) (188) and sterol regulatory element binding proteins (189).

Among these important biomolecules, EPA and DHA are particularly lacking in many contemporary Western dietary regimens, but they are unusual in that a fish-rich diet leads to substantial increases in EPA and DHA. The disparity between a typical Mediterranean diet and Western diet with respect to DHA is not insignificant. The placenta concentrates long-chain polyunsaturated fatty acid metabolites in the fetal circulation (190); preferential conversion of ALA to DHA occurs in women of child-bearing age relative to young men (191–193); and breast milk is a good source of long-chain polyunsaturated fatty acid metabolites that are readily taken up by infants (194,195). Nature clearly intends us to have an adequate DHA status.

Thus, in evolutionary terms, an ancestral diet rich in DHA may explain why contemporary humans are relatively inefficient at synthesizing DHA from ALA. Indeed, it may be that a process similar to that postulated earlier for the loss of *de novo* vitamin C arose because a high intake of n-3 polyunsaturated fatty acids by our ancestors selected against the genetic expression of enzymes responsible for the conversion of ALA to DHA. The possible role of DHA being a selective pressure-driving encephalization, simply by provision of adequate dietary supply of this substrate, has been discussed earlier (92,96).

Under this model, it seems likely that our early African ancestors were as, or more likely to be, fisherman than they were exclusively carnivorous butchers of wild game (196). Indeed, this subject is reviewed in detail by Muskiet et al. (186), who draw attention to the fact that the fish found in the East African Rift Valley lakes are a rich source of AA and DHA compared with their EPA- and DHA-rich counterparts found in more Northern latitudes (197). It has been suggested that a transient drying out of the East African Rift Valley lakes may have been part of the cue that led to early man's expansion out of Africa.

# Chapter 9

# Some Non-Micronutrient Essential and Nonessential Nutrients with Molecular and Possible Evolutionary Impact

## 9.1 LECITHINS

The generic term *lecithin* is used mainly when referring to the body's major phospolipid—phosphatidylcholine. However, it is often used to embrace the four related, major categories of phospholipid. These are phosphatidylcholine, phosphatidylserine, phosphatidylethanolamine, and phosphatidylinositol. The structure is given for these phospholipids in Figure 9.1. The parent generic structure comprises two fatty acid chains esterified to a glycerol moiety, a phosphate group, and a basic component. The basic component is the main variable within the molecular structure of this group of phospholipids.

### 9.1.1 Brain Membranes and Lecthin-Derived Second Messengers

Phosphatidylcholine represents around 50% of the phospholipids in the body and is a critical component of the cell membrane bilayer, being especially abundant in the external membrane leaflet. Its metabolism within the membrane makes it a source of secondary messengers that either activate or repress key cell processes after the release of metabolites into the cytosolic milieu. This inositol membrane lipid signaling system can originate a diverse array of signals that have a huge variety of cell functions. Underpinning this messaging system is phosphatidylinositol (4,5)-bisphosphate (PIB). As an example of the many effects, PIB provides the cofactor for phospolipase D, which hydrolyses phosphatidylcholine

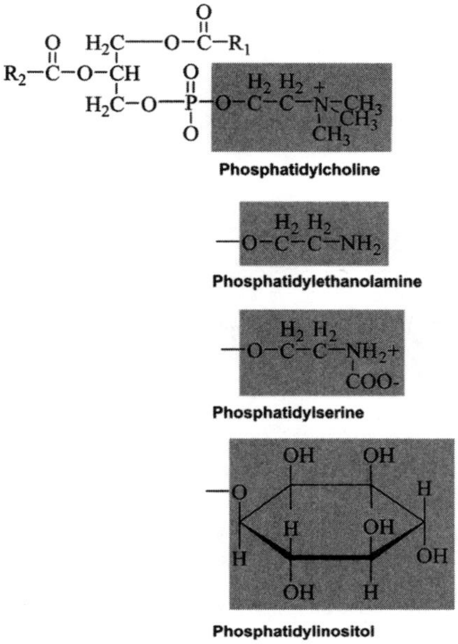

**Figure 9.1.** *Molecular structure of the four major phospholipids.*

to phosphatydic acid, a precursor of diacylglycerol. Diacylglycerol (along with inositol trisphosphate [IP3]) is one of the cells two main secondary messengers and can activate protein kinase C. Activation of protein kinase C (along with secondary messenger activation of the cellular calcium flux by IP3) has a wide range of effects, including secretion, neural activation (including exocytosis), contraction, cell proliferation, and differentiation.

$\alpha$, $\beta$, and $\gamma$ isoforms of protein kinase C have been isolated from the brain, with the $\beta$ isoform being two products derived from alternative splicing of RNA transcripts from the same gene. cDNA cloning has characterized further forms of the protein. $\alpha$ and $\beta$ isoforms of protein kinase C are activated by diacylglycerol and phospholipids in the presence of calcium ions and can be activated by AA. The $\gamma$ isoform is found in nerve tissue, and for this isoform, the activation by AA does not require calcium. Protein kinase C works by preferential phosphorylation of serine or threonine residues on target proteins. Phorbol esters mimic the effects of protein kinase C and are associated with tumor formation, modulating the dynamic between cell differentiation and proliferation, gene expression based on a phorbol ester response element within promoter regions of specific genes, exocytosis, and ionic transport. There are three basic signal transduction mechanisms found within the cell; the diacylglycerol/IP3 system is an example of a second messenger signal transduction pathway. Figure 9.2 shows three major transduction mechanisms as a single schematic.

Dietary phosphatidylcholine provides choline for the brain in its resynthesis of new phosphatidylcholine for cerebral membranes, particularly those of insulating Schwann cells that envelop neuronal axons. Among the good sources of phosphatidylcholine is human breast milk, which actually contains high levels of this phospholipid reflecting its biological purpose—the synthesis of new membranes by the rapidly growing, suckling child. In fact, choline is so abundant that deficiency is extremely uncommon and largely restricted

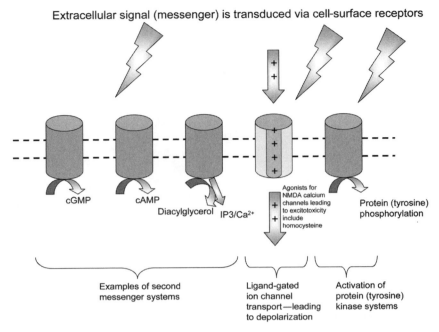

**Figure 9.2.** *Figure showing the various ways in which an extracellular signal can be transduced by cell-surface receptors. The membrane lecthin (phospatidylcholine) derived second messenger is based on diacylglycerol and can activate α and β isoforms of protein kinase C. Protein kinase C works by preferential phosphorylation of serine or threonine residues on target proteins, which modulates cell differentiation and proliferation.*

to rare instances in neonates. This fact not withstanding, it has been determined that dietary phosphatidylcholine ingestion can raise both blood and brain choline levels, and as a consequence stimulate acetylcholine synthesis. Similarly, dietary choline restriction reduces blood and brain acetylcholine. Acetylcholine is a crucial neurotransmitter molecule and is clearly modified by diet. If we consider the brain is 60% lipid, and that unlike many parts of the human anatomy, the human brain develops most rapidly *in utero* and for the first 6 months of life, it seems likely that the lipid content of human breast milk postpartum is an important adjunct to placental nutriture. The other fats of note in the normal functioning of the brain, particularly the early developing brain, are DHA and AA.

Another phospolipid mentioned above is phosphatidylserine, a molecule that may be important in regulating the cell cycle and particularly cell senescence. Phosphatidylserine is restricted to the internal leaflet of the bilayer cell membrane, a process regulated by energy-dependent membrane transport. What is interesting with this molecule is that cells undergoing programmed cell death (apoptosis) rapidly lose this asymmetric distribution of phosphatidylserine between bilayer leaflets. Increasing phosphatidylserine at the outer membrane leaflet during apoptosis provides a phosphatidylserine recognition receptor that signals phagocytosis to occur. This trait has a long evolutionary history, during which time it has been recruited for a range of cellular processes such as blood clotting, and red cell differentiation, as well as membrane fusion.

When you consider the significance of lipids in human development, both in terms of structural elements and in terms of the dynamics of metabolic processes involved in the brain, it is not difficult to see how diet during the earliest phases of the human lifecycle has an important bearing on the well-being of the individual and hence the species as a whole. Given that some of the most important lipids are dietary elements borne out of a food chain with its origins in a marine environment, this has been interpreted by some as a clue to our early origins as was alluded to in Chapter 8.

## 9.2 LIPID-DERIVED FIRST MESSENGERS—THE EICOSANOIDS

As mentioned, AA cannot be synthesized *de novo* and therefore needs to be produced from essential omega-6 series fatty acids such as LLA via chain elongation and desaturation (Figure 8.3). AA along with EPA (omega-3 series) are of biological interest because they serve as precursors for the synthesis of prostaglandins, prostacyclins, leukotrienes, and thromboxanes, which are collectively known as eicosanoids. It is felt that the human dietary requirement for these fatty acids is partially dependent on the important role of eicosanoids within the body. Indeed, the availability of AA determines the rate of synthesis of eicosanoids that cannot be stored in the body.

Prostaglandins, prostacyclin, and thromboxanes are produced from polyunsaturated fatty acids by a specific area of metabolism—the cyclo-oxygenase pathway (Figure 9.3). AA forms the cyclic endoperoxide intermediate prostaglandin $H_2$, which acts as the precursor of the three main prostaglandin series—A, E, and F. The AA-derived prostaglandins are those that have the terminal 2 subscript, indicating that the structure has two double bonds (series-2). Thromboxane $A_2$ and prostacyclin are formed from the cyclic endoperoxide intermediate via isomerization and are local mediators that antagonize one another's actions in terms of the regulation of platelet aggregation and thus blood coagulation (thromboxane $A_2$ stimulates aggregation—prostacyclin inhibits aggregation). They also have an influence on vasoconstriction.

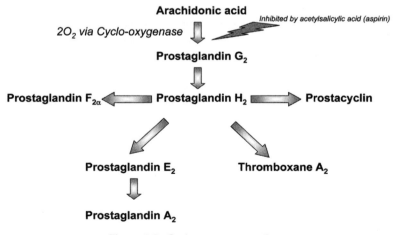

**Figure 9.3.** *Cyclo-oxygenase pathway.*

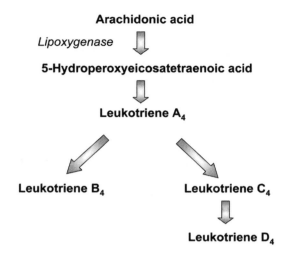

**Figure 9.4.** *Lipoxygenase pathway.*

The leukotrienes are synthesized by a different pathway referred to as the lipoxygenase pathway (Figure 9.4). In this case, AA forms a hydroperoxy fatty acid intermediate in the synthesis of leukotrienes, which cause smooth muscle contracture in the airways of the respiratory tract. Furthermore, leukotriene $B_4$ mediates endothelial cell adhesion and chemotaxis of neutrophils, whereas leukotrenes $C_4$, $D_4$, and $E_4$ are potent mediaters of capilliary vasodilation and permeability.

The balance between omega-3 versus omega-6 series fatty acids is of importance. The n-3 fatty acids act as inhibitors of arachidonic acid (omega-6) metabolism and the related symptoms of an unbalanced production of local lipid mediators. Diets rich in EPA (omega-3) lead to membrane eicosanoid production; EPA competitively inhibits synthesis of leukotrienes from arachidonic acid to produce an anti-inflammatory and immunomodulatory effect; the double-bond structure of EPA produces series-3 prostaglandins, thromboxane, and series-5 leukotrienes, which are metabolically less active than the series-2 prostaglandins, thromboxane, and series-4 leukotriene metabolites of arachidonic acid. Clearly, an important biological synergy is underpinned by the omega-3 to omega-6 fatty acid ratio of our diet.

Hence, one can see how important these essential dietary fatty acids are as precursors of local transitory eicosanoid mediators that play a role in thrombogenic events and conditions such as asthma. In fact, it is now also thought that in high concentrations, eicosanoids are immunosuppressive because of their many effects on lymphocytes and macrophages. Indeed, the altered steroid hormone concentration that initiates childbirth also leads to the production of oxytocin by the pituitary gland and the release of prostaglandin F2$\alpha$, both of which stimulate uterine contraction during childbirth. So significant is this effect that prostaglandins can be used as an abortificient. Prostaglandins also mediate our perception of pain (basis of action of aspirin—see Figure 9.3) and so have far-reaching and significant influence right across the human lifecycle. Clearly, the balance between omega-3 and omega-6 fatty acids is critically important. Humans evolved in an environment that is thought to have provided an omega-3 to omega-6 fatty acid ratio of 1:1. Today, our diets contain too much n-6 and not enough n-3 fatty acids. Infants are likely to be particularly sensitive; it is recommended that the n-6:n-3 ratio (linoleic/linolenic) of infant formula be the same as human milk, i.e., 4:1. Nutritionists are so concerned about this issue that they are considering a revision of the n-6:n-3 ratio from 5 to 2. It has been quoted as being as high as 25 in some modern Western diets. This raises interesting questions regarding the disparity between our early origins, including any link to an ancestral marine-based diet, and our current (and future) fatty acid intake. If the abundance and character of fatty acids played a major role in human evolution, what effect will our current dysfunctional pattern of essential fatty acid intake have on the future of our species?

## 9.3 ISOFLAVONES—GENOMIC AND NONGENOMIC INFLUENCE AT THE ESTROGEN RECEPTOR

Isoflavones are polyphenolic molecules that are variously referred to as flavonoids or phytoestrogens. Phytoestrogens are plant metabolites that can mimic or modulate the natural biological response to endogenous estrogens. The typical Western diet has an isoflavone intake of less than 10 mg/day, whereas in Asia, intake may be 10 times higher, as soy is a major source of food in this geographic region and a rich source of isoflavones. Most isoflavones exist as glycosides or glycones that are conjugated to a glucose moiety. An intestinal glucosidase cleaves the glucose moiety from the glycone to yield an aglycone (Figure 9.5). Aglycones are then absorbed as part of the micelles formed due to the action of the bile acids in the intestinal lumen.

The action of estrogenic isoflavones upon the cell can be as either estrogenic agonists or antagonists. Although this potentially beneficial pharmacologic effect is of interest in relation to tumorgenesis, osteogenesis, and vascular disease, the effect is of special interest in relation to the epithelial cells of reproductive tissue. Ovarian, testicular, and mammary gland

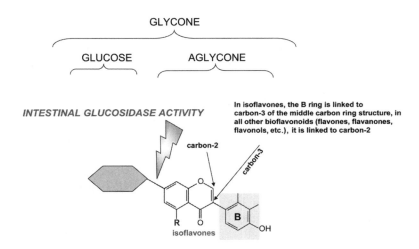

**Enzymatic conversion of glycones to aglycones:**
**Glucosidase within the lumen of the small intestine attacks the glycoside bond in isoflavone glycones to yield an aglycone and glucose moiety**

**Figure 9.5.** *Dietary isoflavones exist as glycosides (glycones) that are conjugated to a glucose residue. An intestinal glucosidase cleaves the glucose moiety from the glycone to yield an aglycone.*

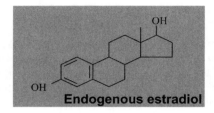

**Figure 9.6.** Molecular similarity between endogenous blood estrogen and two common phytoestrogens.

tissue contain estrogen receptors that are modulated by phytoestrogens. Figure 9.6 shows the similarity between endogenous estradiol and two of the better known isoflavones—daidzein and genistein. Phytoestrogens interact with estrogen receptors in the nucleus where the phytoestrogen–estrogen receptor complex stimulates the nuclear estrogen-response element and transcription (Figure 9.7). In addition to this genomic effect, phytoestrogens may also interact with cell-surface estrogen receptors or influence key cellular enzymes such as topoisomerase 1 that modulate the cell cycle. They may also affect protein phosphorylation and have an antioxidant effect as is observed with bioflavonoids in general. The figure demonstrates the likely cellular genomic and nongenomic effects of isoflavones.

Phytoestrogens are present in many legumes; indeed the effect of this class of molecule upon the reproductive tissue of sheep grazing on clover were one of the first observed effects of phytoestrogens. Australian sheep grazing on clover were found to have decreased fertility. The three major isoflavones are daidzein, glycitein, and genistein, and because of the observed phytoestrogenic effect on reproductive tissue, there has been serious concerns about any similar effect that Soya-based infant formula milk might have on humans—the soybean is a rich source of this nutrient.

It is interesting to ponder whether the use of foods rich in phytoestrogens could ever have had a significant population effect by modifying fertility. It is certainly a bioactive of considerable interest in the area of molecular nutrition.

## 9.4 PHYTIC ACID

Phytic acid (Figure 9.8) is an interesting plant nutrient, which we obtain mostly from grain or soy products. Its ability to bind essential minerals has led to it being thought of as an

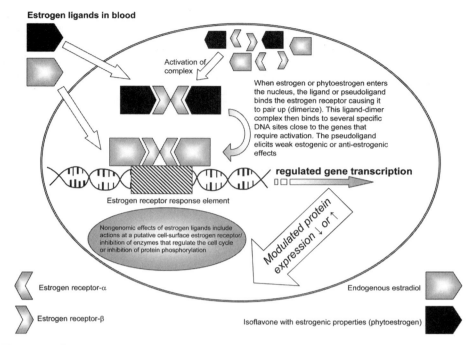

**Figure 9.7.** *Cellular genomic and nongenomic effects of isoflavones. The effects differ according to the type of tissue and the number of estrogen receptors within that tissue. The effect on reproductive tissue is of particular interest and may influence reproductive efficiency.*

anti-nutrient. However, today it is actually considered to have potential anti-tumorigenic properties. Its role in plants is to act as a reservoir of phosphorus and essential divalent mineral cations. When humans ingest phytates, the pH of the gastrointestinal tract is such that, for the most part, phytates do not liberate their bound minerals. In other words, the bioavailability of phytate bound minerals is poor. In the context of reproductive efficiency, the absorption of three key minerals is thought to be impaired by food phytate—these are zinc, iron, and calcium. Given the important role of zinc in particular, it is interesting to

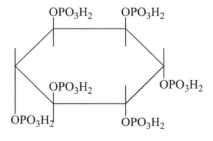

**Phytic acid**

**Figure 9.8.** *Structure of phytic acid, a plant component that can influence the bioavailability of important nutrients like zinc and calcium. The phytate binds mono- and divalent mineral cations via strong ionic interactions.*

consider whether this nutrient might have had any impact on human reproduction in ancestral populations.

The putative anti-cancer effect of phytic acid is thought to relate to the fact that it is an inositol phosphate, and hence that it may have a second messenger role via mechanisms that were alluded to earlier. Inositol phosphates derived from phytic acid and released from membranes may therefore act as key metabolic switches.

# Chapter 10

# Natural Food Toxins and the Human Diet

Clearly, the availability of food is an important determinant of human survival if not evolution. Quite early in our prehistory, we learned that heat treatment could detoxify the poisonous constituents within potential food sources. Over the subsequent years we evolved better ways of processing foods and, thus, increased the repertoire of foods available for consumption.

To place a chronological context to the art of detoxifying food sources, 15,000 years ago, the early inhabitants of the Australian continent had already mastered the skill of processing out toxic compounds from the nutrient-rich cycad nut. Depending on the species, the seeds might be cooked, crushed into flour, and then the toxins washed out in running water for several days before being used to make bread. Some species of poisonous cycad were also used by Australian Aborigines to assist in the healing process, as well as for food. An example of a cycad species used by Aborigines for both healing and food is the Queensland cycad *Cycas media*.

## 10.1 DIETARY ZOOTOXINS

One of the major organ foods of concern regarding dietary toxins is liver. The liver can accumulate bile acids such as cholic acid, deoxycholic, acid, and taurocholic acid (cholic acid being the most toxic). Preparations of dried bear liver have been used as a traditional medicine for many centuries, and the basis for this unethical pharmaceutical product is the tranquilizing and analgesic properties of the endogenous bile acids. Taken in large quantity, the liver may therefore have a toxic effect, although clearly any impact on the foraging activities of early man is difficult to assess. Another compound found in the liver is also toxic in high concentrations: Excess vitamin A derived from polar bear or oily fish livers has

*Molecular Nutrition and Genomics: Nutrition and the Ascent of Humankind*, by Mark Lucock
Copyright © 2007 John Wiley & Sons, Inc.

## Spectrum of effects of preformed vitamin A

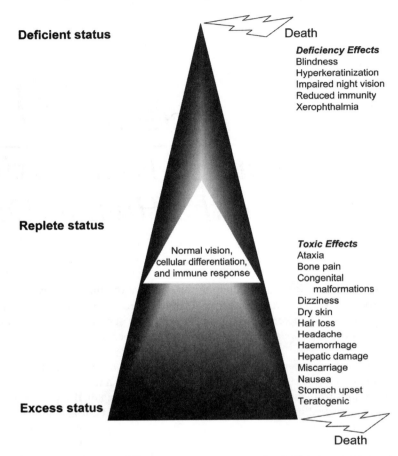

**Figure 10.1.** *Preformed vitamin A (not carotenoid derived provitamin A) has a spectrum of effects that in extreme cases (i.e., too much or too little) can lead to death. In particular, excess vitamin A derived from polar bear or oily fish livers has been associated with serious clinical conditions.*

been associated with several clinical conditions such as skin irritation and bleeding, bone pain, drowsiness, headache, and ultimately death. Clearly, some dietary essentials have a spectrum of activity that at the upper limits can lead to toxicity, despite our obligate need for them. In this respect, preformed vitamin A is the classic example. As mentioned earlier, given its critical role in developmental regulation, excess vitamin A has been associated with neuronal malformations, and the vitamin is considered to be teratogenic. Figure 10.1 shows the spectrum of effects that different planes of vitamin A nutriture can elicit.

Our early diet may well have been based on marine resources, a form of food with notable issues relating to potential toxicity (Figure 10.2). Indeed, despite the issues associated with excess liver intake, terrestrial animal foods have far fewer toxicity problems than do marine animals.

## Some examples of marine food toxins

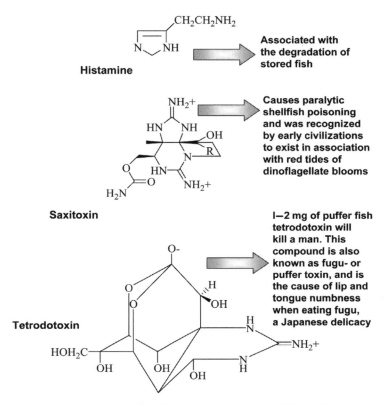

**Histamine** — Associated with the degradation of stored fish

**Saxitoxin** — Causes paralytic shellfish poisoning and was recognized by early civilizations to exist in association with red tides of dinoflagellate blooms

**Tetrodotoxin** — I–2 mg of puffer fish tetrodotoxin will kill a man. This compound is also known as fugu- or puffer toxin, and is the cause of lip and tongue numbness when eating fugu, a Japanese delicacy

**Figure 10.2.** *Molecular structure of three different marine toxins, which exhibit a large spectrum of effect from histamine tainting through to the extreme neurotoxicity caused by puffer fish tetrodotoxin. Our ancestors recognized the potential toxic nature of red tides that were the result of algal blooms, as the phenomenon had such a profound effect on a major food resource.*

The microbial degradation of stored fish can lead to bacterial decarboxylation of histidine and hence formation of histamine. Histamine can accumulate at high concentrations in stored fish before the sensory cue for detecting tainted odors cuts in. The gastrointestinal, neurologic, and sensory effects of this toxicity may be due to a synergy between histamine and polyamines in the contaminated fish, and generally it wears off quickly, with death being a rare outcome.

Most people recognize the potential toxic effect of shellfish, which is due to the poisonous substance saxitoxin. Saxitoxin induces what is commonly called "paralytic shellfish poisoning" and is associated with extensive dinoflagellate blooms. This algal phenomenon is often referred to as a "red tide". Early civilizations were often well aware of the clear-cut association between the development of a red tide and saxitoxin-contaminated shell fish that could precipitate illness. The condition is largely confined to areas outside the 30 degrees of latitude above and below the equator. Crustaceans can also accumulate toxins, some as a consequence of living in an area with a red tide.

Other marine toxins of note include tetrodotoxin from puffer fish, tetramine and pyropheophorbide from marine mollusks, and ciguatoxin, which causes ichthyotoxism or fish poisoning. There can be little doubt that tetrodotoxin is the best known of these toxins, probably in recognition of its role in the Japanese delicacy fugu, which is carefully prepared by Sushi chefs licensed by the Japanese government. However, tetrodotoxin is an acutely potent neurotoxin that leads to voltage-gated sodium channel blockade on the surface of nerve membranes and causes a regular plethora of deaths each year.

**Table 10.1. Some examples of food phytotoxins.**

| Source (Examples Only) | Bioactive Molecule(s) | Mode of Action | Biological Effect |
|---|---|---|---|
| Cassava root Cycad nut | **Cyanogenic glycosides**, i.e., amygdalin and linamarin | Cyanide toxicity leading to inhibition of the mitochondrial respiratory chain | Cytochrome oxidase inhibition, tropical ataxic neuropathy, tropical amblyopia (destruction of optic nerve) |
| Cruciferous plants (cabbage family) | **Goitrogens** i.e., thiocyanate and goitrin formed from glucosinolates | Thyroid gland enlargement: goitrin inhibits thyroxine synthesis, thiocyanates inhibit thyroid tissue uptake of iodine | In areas where milk forms a primary source of iodine, cattle fed on goitrogen-rich feed may produce iodine-depleted milk, and exacerbate goiter (enlarged thyroid gland) formation following human consumption |
| Vicia fava beans | **Aglycones** divicine and isouramil (corresponding glycosides are vicine and convicine) | Aglycones precipitate favism, which may be linked to altered glucose and glutathione metabolism | Fatality rare, but causes general malaise, abdominal discomfort, and fever. Kidneys can fail, but recovery is usual after 48 hours |
| Legumes | **Lectins** | May reduce intestinal absorption of nutrients and impair barrier to bacterial infection | Possible anti-nutrient |
| Pea species of the genus *Lathyrus* | Possibly caused by **$\beta$-N-oxalyl-L-$\alpha,\beta$-diaminopropionic acid** | Causes lathyrism—specifically neurolathyrism in humans. May influence glutamate-related neurotransmission in the brain | Progressive paralysis of lower limbs with associated muscle rigidity and generalized weakness. Commonly associated with consumption of *Lathyrus sativus* |
| Various plants producing pyrrolizidine alkaloids that may pass into the human food chain or be used as herbal remedies | **Pyrrolizidine alkaloids** | Mutagenic | May cause cancer. Many other natural mutagens are found in plant foods, i.e., some flavonoids |
| Calibar bean; species of the genus *Solanum*, i.e., potatoes, tomatoes, egg plant | **Glycoalkaloid—anticholinesterases**: Physostigmine (calabar bean), solanine (*Solanum sp*) | Anticholinesterase activity | Variable effect—green potatoes cause gut pain, nausea, sickness, and difficulty breathing. Physostigmine affect is very profound and is the basis of carbamate insecticides |

**Food cyanogenic glycosides**

Amygdalin

Cyanide groups that confer
toxicity to cyanogenic glycosides

Linamarin

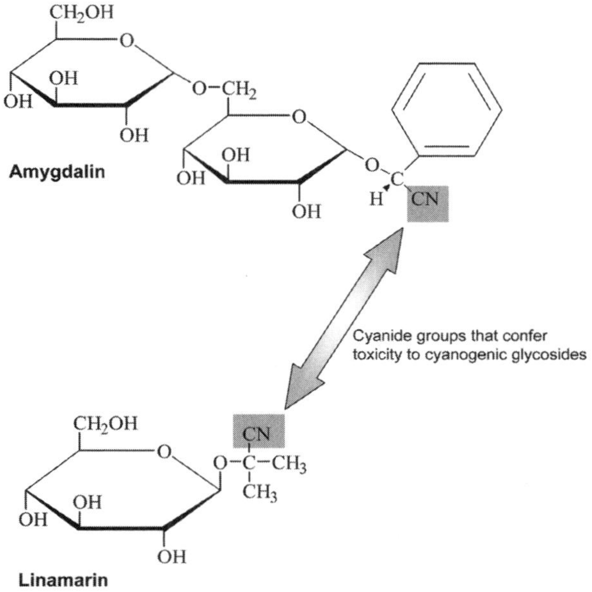

**Figure 10.3.** *Figure gives examples of two cyanogenic glycosides found in food that can lead to cyanide toxicity. Cyanide is extremely toxic and binds to the ferric ion of mitochondrial cytochrome oxidase inhibiting cellular respiration—this is the well-known acute effect of cyanide poisoning. The chronic effects— i.e., of linamarin ingestion from cassava—include tropical ataxic neuropathy and tropical amblyopia.*

## 10.2 DIETARY PHYTOTOXINS

Human dietary selection has been refined over the millennia to exclude consumption of excessively toxic plant species. Plants are a cocktail of chemicals, many designed to prevent their consumption by conferring toxicity. This may be reflected in reduced palatability, or it may manifest itself by producing a far more lethal molecular milieu.

This is by its very nature a large area of study, with many categories of phytotoxin to consider. To simplify the subject, Table 10.1 shows some brief information on selected phytotoxins. Figure 10.3 illustrates the molecular structure of two phytotoxins that confer cyanide toxicity. Linamarin is of concern as it is found in the staple tropical food— cassava.

# Chapter *11*

# *Nutrigenomics*

## 11.1 WHAT IS NUTRIGENOMICS?

I provided a definition of nutritional genetics and nutrigenomics earlier. Most of the information detailed in this book is hung on a framework of one or the other of these important areas. However, although my theme throughout this book has been on the role of nutrition in human evolution, scientists around the world have tackled these important areas largely to help understand and attenuate human disease and suffering.

Muller and Kersten (198) describe nutrigenomics as the application of high-throughput genomics tools in nutrition research. With this in mind, one can immediately see how important the Human Genome Project has been in illuminating the molecular signature of those genes that have particular relevance to our diet. The Human Genome Project has provided the world's scientists with enormous amounts of accessible bioinformatics data. In the West, the Internet has given consumers the same level of access to information for attaining nutritional optima that maintains health and well-being. Increased awareness by consumers on matters of diet and health has helped to forge today's marketing strategies. Already we are seeing the public responding to personal nutrigenomic information, and this is a trend that is only going to increase. Although this obviates any evolutionary forces that may be at work, it is likely to have profound future effects on population health.

Two caveats may be added to this: (1) Market forces can be used to distort reality. I worry about products that are sold with a singular marketing ploy that oversells a nutrient's health benefits. There are several products with health benefit upsides that may possibly also have some downsides. It is always best to emphasize moderation and balance when talking dietary regimes. (2) Some (not so small) sectors of the population are slow to adapt to public health messages.

In essence, nutrigenomics considers dietary components as signals detected by cellular sensing systems that transduce these into the expression of proteins that regulate metabolite levels (Figure 11.1). Nutrigenomics therefore looks at how nutrients influence the cell's homeostatic signature. Inherent in this global perspective is the search for genes and their

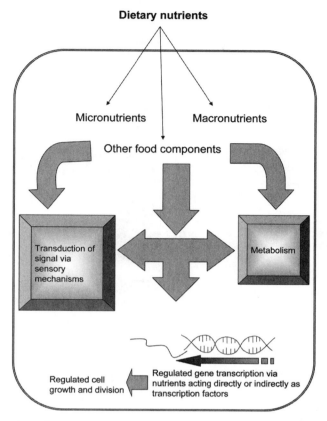

**Figure 11.1.** Simple scheme showing nutrigenomic aspects of cellular function.

polymorphic forms that predispose us to disease, but that can be modified in their effect by dietary nutrients.

Earlier, Table 3.1 showed a range of important micronutrient–gene interactions that are important elements in the study of nutrigenomics. Figure 11.2 shows some products that are encoded by vitamin A and D responsive genes. Macronutrients are also important and can similarly act through transcription factor pathways that mediate nutrient–gene interactions (see Figure 11.3):

Carbohydrates such as glucose interact with transcription factors like upstream stimulatory factor, sterol-responsive-element binding protein, and carbohydrate responsive binding protein. Fats like cholesterol also act with sterol-responsive-element binding protein, and with the liver X receptor and farnesoid X receptor (bile salt receptor [FXR]). Fatty acids interact with PPARs and hepatocyte nuclear factor among others, and amino acids interact with CCAAT/enhancer-binding protein.

Transcription factors are the most important mechanism by which nutrients influence the expression of genes. To place this in context, there are 48 members of the nuclear hormone receptor superfamily of transcription factors. Many of these have already been mentioned: PPARs, RAR, RXR, VDR, LXR, and FXR.

Without doubt, the future challenge in nutrigenomics is to elucidate further nutrient-modulated molecular pathways and determine downstream effects. Only then will we be

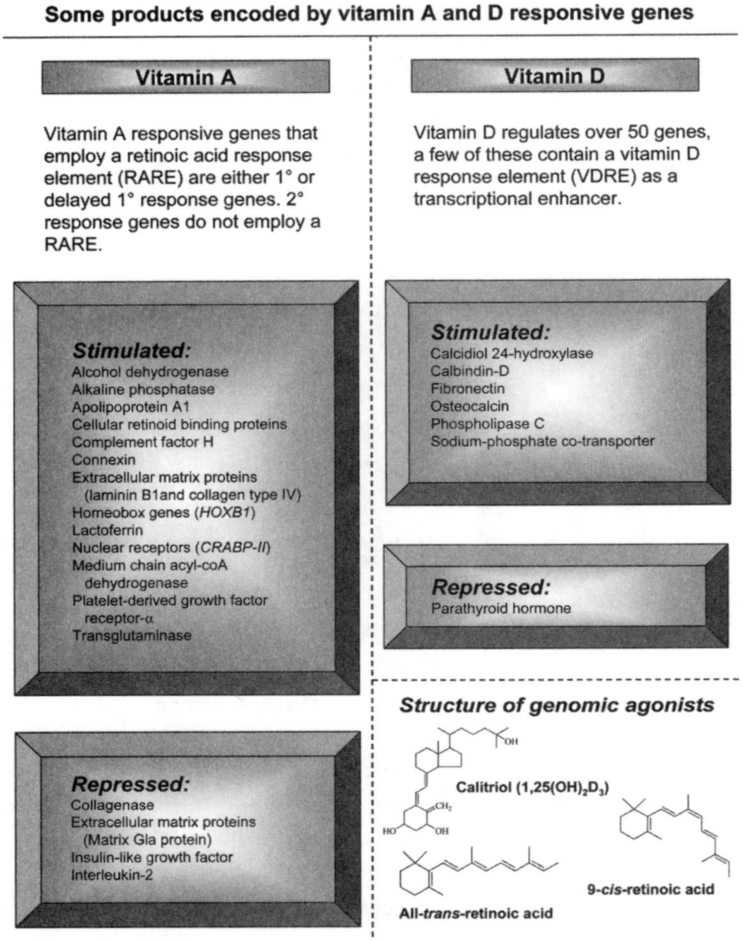

**Some products encoded by vitamin A and D responsive genes**

| Vitamin A | Vitamin D |
|---|---|
| Vitamin A responsive genes that employ a retinoic acid response element (RARE) are either 1° or delayed 1° response genes. 2° response genes do not employ a RARE. | Vitamin D regulates over 50 genes, a few of these contain a vitamin D response element (VDRE) as a transcriptional enhancer. |

**Stimulated:**
Alcohol dehydrogenase
Alkaline phosphatase
Apolipoprotein A1
Cellular retinoid binding proteins
Complement factor H
Connexin
Extracellular matrix proteins
  (laminin B1and collagen type IV)
Homeobox genes (*HOXB1*)
Lactoferrin
Nuclear receptors (*CRABP-II*)
Medium chain acyl-coA
  dehydrogenase
Platelet-derived growth factor
  receptor-α
Transglutaminase

**Stimulated:**
Calcidiol 24-hydroxylase
Calbindin-D
Fibronectin
Osteocalcin
Phospholipase C
Sodium-phosphate co-transporter

**Repressed:**
Parathyroid hormone

**Repressed:**
Collagenase
Extracellular matrix proteins
  (Matrix Gla protein)
Insulin-like growth factor
Interleukin-2

**Structure of genomic agonists**

Calitriol (1,25(OH)$_2$D$_3$)

9-*cis*-retinoic acid

All-*trans*-retinoic acid

**Figure 11.2.** Examples of some products that are encoded by vitamin A and D responsive genes.

able to comprehend the true influence of nutrition on human well-being. When that time arrives, human molecular nutrition will reach full maturity as a life sciences discipline.

## 11.2 GENETIC BUFFERING UNDERPINS NUTRIGENOMIC RELATIONSHIPS

Random or stochastic variations in the natural environment such as food availability and mutagenic agents confound life processes. However, despite the many factors that impact on the fidelity of DNA, and orchestration of our metabolome, our biological systems remain extraordinarily stable.

The balance between phenotypic stability and instability is regulated by genetic buffering mechanisms that interact with environmental variables. These buffering mechanisms are an integral part of the human nutrigenomic profile and include gene duplication mechanisms, the complex regulatory mesh of epistatic (gene–gene) interactions, and protein–protein interactions that confer molecular stability in a relatively nonspecific manner. More obvious

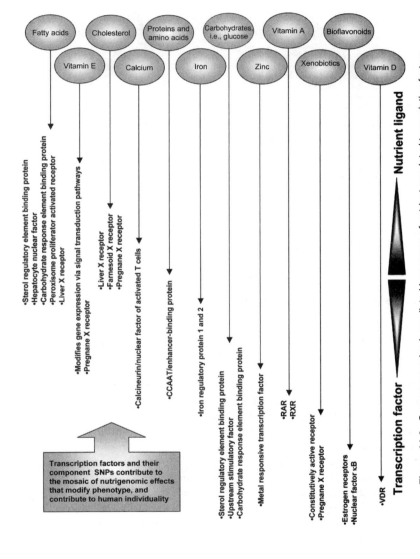

**Figure 11.3.** Gene expression is mediated by a range of nutrient-regulated transcription factors.

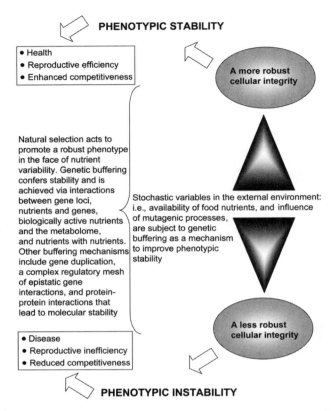

**PHENOTYPIC STABILITY**

- Health
- Reproductive efficiency
- Enhanced competitiveness

A more robust cellular integrity

Natural selection acts to promote a robust phenotype in the face of nutrient variability. Genetic buffering confers stability and is achieved via interactions between gene loci, nutrients and genes, biologically active nutrients and the metabolome, and nutrients with nutrients. Other buffering mechanisms include gene duplication, a complex regulatory mesh of epistatic gene interactions, and protein-protein interactions that lead to molecular stability

Stochastic variables in the external environment: i.e., availability of food nutrients, and influence of mutagenic processes, are subject to genetic buffering as a mechanism to improve phenotypic stability

A less robust cellular integrity

- Disease
- Reproductive inefficiency
- Reduced competitiveness

**PHENOTYPIC INSTABILITY**

*Figure 11.4.* The balance between phenotypic outcomes with respect to nutrition and genetic buffering.

nutritional interactions clearly also exist between many nutrients and a wide variety of genes, biologically active food-derived molecules and the metabolome, and nutrients with nutrients.

When these buffering mechanisms fail, a less robust cellular integrity ensues, leading to phenotypic instability. This could mean a reduced reproductive potential, a less competitive individual with respect to sequestering food, and/or the occurrence of disease. Figure 11.4 shows a schematic of the balance between phenotypic outcomes with respect to nutrition and genetic buffering.

It is relatively easy to construct a simple mapping of nutritionally relevant interactions that lead to a particular phenotype if one limits the mapping to a fairly small area of the interactome. For example, dietary folate is required for *de novo* methionine biosynthesis (i.e., DNA methylation regulated gene expression and hundreds of other biomethylations), nucleotide formation (production of thymine for the elaboration of DNA), amino acid interconversions, and the lowering of athero-, neuro-, and embryotoxic homocysteine. Many proteins that facilitate folate-dependent one-carbon transfer reactions, or act as folate carriers, or that simply lead to the addition or removal of polyglutamyl tails that are required for cellular retention/reactivity, are encoded by common polymorphic genes. These variant folate genes do not work in isolation; (199) epistasis occurs with significant interactions. For example, within the potentially deleterious C677T-MTHFR–TT genotype, four other folate SNPs (A1298C-MTHFR, G80A-reduced folate carrier [G80A-RFC], A2756G-methionine synthase [A2756G-MS], and A66G-methionine synthase reductase [A66G-MSR]) seem to determine the balance between homocysteine transsulphuration to cysteine and folate-related homocysteine remethylation to methionine (199). It is already well recognized that a limited permutation of C677T- and A1298C-MTHFR genotypes is possible—three or four mutant alleles within this haplotype are extremely rare if at all possible. The MS and MSR genes that exist as common variants have a close interaction because their gene products are dependent proteins, which along with vitamin $B_{12}$, interact in the *de novo* biosynthesis of methionine and the regeneration of tetrahydrofolate for nucleotide biosynthesis. In this reaction, MS-bound vitamin $B_{12}$ cycles between methylcobalamin and cob(I)alamin forms of vitamin $B_{12}$. As the cob(I)alamin form is susceptible to oxidation, leading to an inactive cob(II)alamin form of the enzyme, MSR in concert with S-adenosylmethionine is required to salvage this molecular species for further catalytic cycling (200, 201). The occurrence (over-representation within a clinical phenotype) of these and other similar folate SNPs is now associated with risk for several developmental and degenerative conditions. Many of these SNPs also have functional metabolic consequences ascribed to them that are likely to influence the robustness of the clinical phenotype—sometimes for the better, sometimes for the worse.

In addition, vitamins C, $B_2$, and $B_6$ also play important roles in folate metabolism in a similar manner to $B_{12}$. That is, they exhibit significant direct and indirect nutrient–nutrient interactions with respect to folate: Secretion of vitamin C into the gastric lumen aids the bioavailability of reduced dietary folate, $B_2$ is a cofactor for MTHFR, and $B_6$ is required as a cofactor for serinehydroxymethyl transferase (SHMT) and cystathionine $\beta$-synthase (C$\beta$S). Therefore, both $B_2$ and $B_6$ impact upon the interconversion of the various pathway specific one-carbon forms of folate.

Folate, and as a consequence, $B_{12}$ $B_2$, and possibly $B_6$ also provide a good example of direct nutrient–gene interactions. On the one hand, folate provides the one-carbon unit for conversion of uracil to thymine needed in the elaboration of DNA, and it provides methyl groups for gene expression, which is a direct general effect of diet upon the human transcriptome. On the other hand, folate SNPs interact with folate status to influence risk for a variety of diseases and reproductive health. In the latter case it would seem that the abundance of dietary folate may even select folate-related SNPs in the early embryo and offer a survival advantage under the prevailing nutritional environment (25, 37).

A very clear nutrient–gene interaction is given by G80A-RFC. This common folate SNP in the reduced folate carrier protein (RFC) is responsible for subtly altering the cellular uptake of the proteins major folyl ligand-5-methyltetrahydrofolate (202). RFC is responsible for the uptake of folate from the jejunum (203) and the subsequent translocation of this trace nutrient across the membranes of a variety of cells (204, 205).

This SNP at position 80 (exon 2) of the RFC gene is represented by the substitution of a guanine for an adenine (G80A RFC), and it leads to an arginine replacing a histidine in the expressed carrier protein. The functional effect of the expressed polymorphic receptor protein is the altered assimilation of folate from dietary sources into red cells (erythrocytes) (202), which is a process that occurs during erythropoiesis in the bone marrow. Interestingly, RFC is particularly abundant in tissues that have a high folate requirement, i.e., reproductive tissues. This means that G80A-RFC may potentially influence reproductive efficacy, although this speculative possibility remains to be proven.

Although modern data sets within nutrigenomics and the whole "omics" revolution tend to have very high dimensionality, leading to a clear need for *in silico* modeling of such systems biology "omic" supersets, it is possible to focus in on one area and to examine how overall genetic variability and selected nutrient–nutrient interactions might influence cell biology and, hence, phenotype. Using the folate variant genes described above, Figure 11.5

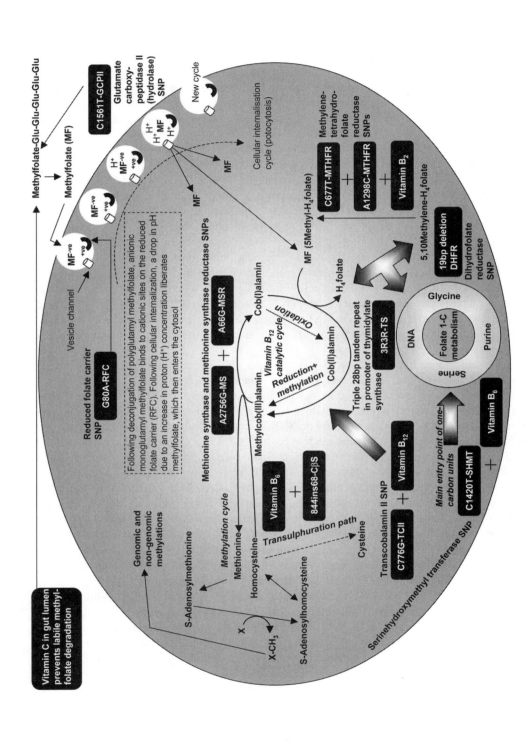

**Figure 11.5.** *With reference to a selected area of folate metabolism, this simplified figure shows how overall genetic variability and selected nutrient–nutrient interactions might influence cell biology and, hence, phenotype. The overall pattern of the genotypes shown (others SNPs exist but are not given), and availability of dependent nutrients, even within this small area of metabolism will modify an individual's potential phenotype with respect to developmental and degenerative disease risk. C677T-MTHFR is the classic example, but others include a common dihydrofolate reductase 19–base pair deletion allele that acts as a risk factor for preterm delivery (206), whereas A2756G-MS and G80A-RFC modify risk of developing a life-threatening blood clot. C677T-MTHFR and A66G-MSR can act together to increase risk for Down syndrome, whereas folate, $B_{12}$, C677T-MTHFR, A1298C-MTHFR, and A66G-MSR have all been implicated in the etiology of neural tube defects. Furthermore, the biological availability and/or effectiveness of vitamin $B_{12}$ and vitamin C may be compromised in atrophic gastritis, and thus may have a secondary impact on folate metabolism. The points of impact and permutations of potential interaction and hence the overall spectrum of variability, even in this small area of metabolism, are clearly immense. Expand the area of interest, and one can readily appreciate that nutrigenomics encompasses a very high dimensionality, leading to the clear need for* in silico *modeling of systems biology "omic" supersets.*

shows a simple mapping to illustrate the bespoke architecture within metabolic pathways. One can liken this mapping to a town plan. As an example, if one assumes that SNPs exist to benefit the organism under certain circumstances, one can envision a simple parallel. Think of a very busy road that has 100 accidents within a notorious one-mile stretch each year. The council then installs a series of speed bumps (sleeping policemen) and chicanes that slow the traffic up. As a consequence, the number of accidents drops to 20 per year. If one thinks of each speed measure as a SNP, one can see how an SNP might confer benefit. One can similarly draw the parallel of diversionary measures to improve traffic flow where access to key urban facilities may be limited. In this context, consider the MTHFR protein. The C677T-MTHFR variant may slow one-carbon unit "traffic" flow to methionine synthesis, but providing overall folate status is good, it leads to a diversion, and hence enhanced one-carbon unit "traffic" flow into thymine, one of the building blocks of DNA. By regulating metabolic traffic in this way, SNPs aid phenotypic stability. One can similarly view nutrient cofactors that act in synergy with folate as payment that has to be provided at tollbooths that permit onward passage of one-carbon units. Without wanting to appear trite, the town plan analogy has much to commend it.

# Chapter 12

# *The Evolution of Protein Function*

As explained earlier, due to the triplet base encryption within codons, mutations that lead to altered code encryption will yield a different amino acid in the expressed protein. Such mutational changes in the amino acid sequence of a protein are a natural part of the evolutionary process. However, such mutations would only be tolerated if (1) their effect on the structural integrity and functional role of the protein was neutral, or (2) their effect was beneficial in a way that could augment stability and/or function (Figures 12.1 and 12.2). Clearly, with this paradigm, any negative mutational change would be eradicated by natural selection.

If we consider the three-dimensional structure of a protein, the evolution of change to such structures is inherently slow for amino acids at the structural core, but considerably more rapid at amino acid residues that are exposed on the protein surface. At the core, mutational changes in amino acid residues are far more likely to influence structural integrity than are similar changes at the proteins surface. The major criterion for surface residues is that they are hydrophilic, and so change here is potentially less detrimental and more likely to be the subject of evolutionary forces. The tertiary three-dimensional structure of a protein is determined by the organization of secondary structural elements ($\alpha$-helices and $\beta$-sheets). This secondary structural organization tends to pack together in a manner that renders the core hydrophobic and is interconnected via polypeptide chains that are referred to as "loops," which tend to be hydrophilic and lay at the protein surface. It is these loop structures at the surface that are subject to a greater rate of evolutionary change than the other secondary structural elements. Similarly, membrane-spanning proteins such as G-proteins evolve slower in the intramembrane spanning elements than in the loops that connect them and that extend beyond the membrane surface.

It is therefore perhaps unsurprising that the structure of a protein is conserved despite dramatic evolutionary changes to the sequence. Hence, many proteins exist with similar structure, but with very different functions. Equally, substantial sequence differences

**Intramolecular factors that contribute to protein stability**

Development of:
Hydrophobic interaction forces
Electrostatic interactions (*based on charge*)
London and van der Waals forces
Hydrogen bonding
Above noncovalent forces promote protein folding
    and stability

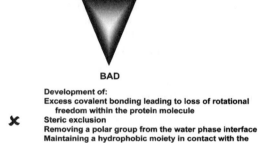

GOOD

A protein–ligand interaction is based on the equilibrium between
favoarable and an unfavoarable structural possibility within the
molecular scaffolding of the protein

BAD

Development of:
Excess covalent bonding leading to loss of rotational
    freedom within the protein molecule
Steric exclusion
Removing a polar group from the water phase interface
Maintaining a hydrophobic moiety in contact with the
    water phase interface

**Figure 12.1.** *A range of intramolecular factors contribute to protein stability and, hence, function: Protein–ligand interactions are based on the evolution of an equilibrium between favorable and unfavorable structural possibilities within the molecular scaffolding of the protein.*

can exist, but functional similarity is retained: Myoglobin, leghemoglobin, and hemoglobin polypeptide chains all assist in oxygen transport by a similar mechanism and have a common ancestral protein but have a sequence homology below 20%. Clearly, although sequence homology has been lost, structures remain similar. Thus, both sequence and three-dimensional structure are extremely important in determining key evolutionary relationships.

**Serine residue**

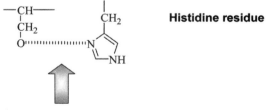

**Histidine residue**

Example of a common hydrogen bond found within proteins,
which contributes to overall protein stability

**Figure 12.2.** *Hydrogen bonds are one intramolecular force that is found within proteins, which contributes to the overall molecular stability and function.*

Certain amino acid residues have a tendency to be conserved through evolution because they are critical to structural integrity and include cysteine, which is needed for the maintenance of disulphide bridges, glycine due to its conformational flexibility, and proline due to its ability to produce *cis-* and *trans*-conformations.

Gene duplication is a potential mechanism for the development of a new protein function. Another mechanism is the development of an interaction between different domains within multidomain proteins. This mechanism will evolve a far more complex protein function than existed in the ancestral protein.

One of the best-known programs for viewing three-dimensional protein structures to evaluate structural interactions is RasMol.

If an SNP changes the encoded amino acid sequence within the mRNA transcript, it is referred to as a nonsynonymous nucleotide substitution. If a nonsynonymous nucleotide substitution is conservative, it is likely that the physicochemical properties of the amino acid substituent do not differ from the wildtype amino acid, and hence, the SNP will be silent—i.e., not affect the phenotype. However, nonconservative, nonsynonymous nucleotide substitutions do alter the physicochemical properties of the protein and, hence, modify phenotype. The common C677T-MTHFR polymorphism discussed earlier results in an alanine-to-valine substitution within this key cellular enzyme protein (MTHFR (A222V) and stems from the alanine GCC codon being altered to a valine GTC codon. This C-to-T nucleotide substitution provides an excellent example of a nonconservative, nonsynonymous nucleotide substitution in which the expressed protein alters phenotype.

# Chapter *13*

# *Leading Edge Laboratory Tools in Nutrigenomics and Human Evolutionary Studies*

## 13.1 DENATURING HPLC

Denaturing high-performance liquid chromatography (dHPLC) is a relatively new technique for detecting heteroduplex DNAs. The method works by subjecting two amplicons (amplified PCR products—see below) consisting of double-stranded DNAs that differ in one nucleotide to an annealing temperature that forms hetero- and homoduplexes that can be separated by a variant form of HPLC. The technique is excellent at detecting new and potentially interesting SNPs in candidate genes, a discriminatory process that is achieved using statistical cluster analysis. See Figure 13.1 showing a dHPLC system.

## 13.2 DNA SEQUENCING

The information contained within the human blueprint for life can be read using DNA sequencing technology. The major advance in this approach came when Fred Sanger developed the dideoxy chain termination method, work that led to his second Nobel Prize. The "Sanger" method for DNA sequencing permits stretches of 500–800 DNA bases at a time to be read.

In the modern laboratory, automated instrumentation controlled by computers allows vast amounts of data to be accumulated. A sequence reaction is performed using dideoxynucleotide triphosphates (ddNTPs) that are labeled with different colored dyes.

DNA is copied by DNA polymerase, and ddNTPs in the reaction mixture cause random termination of DNA polymerization. This produces a ladder of DNA fragments, which can be detected by laser excitation as they migrate through a polyacrylamide gel.

*Molecular Nutrition and Genomics: Nutrition and the Ascent of Humankind*, by Mark Lucock
Copyright © 2007 John Wiley & Sons, Inc.

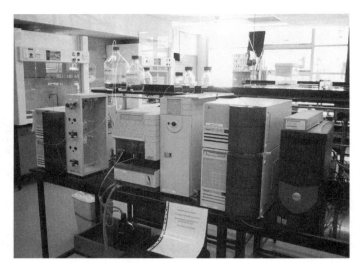

**Figure 13.1.** *A dHPLC designed for the detection of new and potentially interesting SNPs in candidate genes.*

This technique has been used to sequence entire genomes that are billions of base pairs long, albeit in bite-sized portions around 500 base pairs in length.

## 13.3 NUCLEIC ACID MICROCHIP TECHNIQUES

Nucleic acid microchips permit the analysis of thousands of genes simultaneously and in a very rapid manner. In essence, these chips, which are often referred to as DNA microarrays, are minute wafers to which a variety of oligonucleotides have been attached in a highly ordered array using fine computer guided jets or photolithography. Either DNA or RNA from cells or physiologic fluids can be hybridized to these microarrays. The DNA deposited on the array is known as the "probe," whereas the cellular nucleic acids under investigation that hybridize to the probes are known as "targets."

This technique can be used to study gene expression; in which case, the arrays are composed of probes that describe a range of specific genes. Clearly with this approach the targets are mRNA transcripts (normally after conversion to a fluorescent cDNA by the enzyme reverse transcriptase). Using this approach one can study gene expression under variable sets of conditions, and study the factors that ultimately lead to different proteins being expressed—this tool is valuable in nutrigenomics. The array of oligonucleotide probes indicates expression by a fluorescent signal within the array grid. The fluorescent probe thus provides a unique signature for that specific gene of interest.

DNA microarrays are also extremely important for determining (scoring) SNPs. The probes are synthons of short oligonucleotides that contain the polymorphic base (synthons are manufactured to contain different substitutions of the base of interest in order to deduce the nature of the target). The arrangement of the array is such that hybridization between probe and target provides the necessary information to genotype an individual. Fidelity is assured because stringent hybridization conditions are applied. Up to 2000 SNPs can be scored on some microarrays.

## 13.4 THE POLYMERASE CHAIN REACTION

The polymerase chain reaction (PCR) is a technique that is used to amplify a sequence of DNA. Amplified segments of DNA are known as amplicons. The amplification process involves using a short (20–25 bases) pair of oligonucleotide primers that are each complementary to one end of the target DNA sequence. Thus, one primer is "sense or forward," and one is "antisense or reverse."

The following table shows the primer sequences for detecting two common SNPs of 5,10MTHFR:

**Table 13.1. Forward and reverse primer sequences for detecting two common SNPs of 5,10MTHFR. The primers are used in the amplification process and are typical in using a short (20–25 bases) pair of oligonucleotides that are each complementary to one end of the target DNA sequence. The two primers in each set are extended toward one another by Taq-polymerase in a three-step cycle involving denaturation, primer annealing, and nucleotide polymerization.**

| Primer Sequences for two common 5,10MTHFR SNPs | |
| --- | --- |
| Forward primer | Reverse primer |
| **C677T MTHFR**   TGA AGG AGA AGG TGT CTG CGG GA | AGG ACG GTG CGG TGA GAG TG |
| **A1298C MTHFR**   CTT TGG GGA GCT GAA GGA CTA CTA C | CAC TTT GTG ACC ATT CCG GTT TG |

The primers are extended toward each other by a DNA polymerase that is heat stable and originates from an organism that has adapted to life in thermal springs. This organism, *Thermophilus aquaticus*, gives its name to the enzyme Taq-polymerase. Taq-polymerase is thus extremely heat resistant at temperatures that permit DNA denaturation, and this is what allows the laboratory amplification of DNA to occur.

The sense and antisense primers are extended toward one another by Taq-polymerase in a three-step reaction cycle that involves (1) denaturation, (2) primer annealing, and (3) nucleotide polymerization (elongation).

The reaction cycle typically consists of a 95°C step to denature duplex DNA into single-stranded DNA, an annealing step of around 55°C for annealing (binding of primers), and a 72°C elongation step (see Figure 13.2).

The following table again uses the two common SNPs of 5,10MTHFR as examples to illustrate how the time-temperature coefficient for cycling is varied very slightly to provide optimal amplicon synthesis. These conditions are used in the author's laboratory.

The reaction mixture that is required for PCR must include dNTPs, magnesium, forward and reverse primers, buffer, Taq-polymerase, and the DNA template, perhaps extracted from blood or cheek cells.

In theory, only one target DNA template molecule is needed for amplification, although in practice, many template molecules are usually present within a PCR reaction mixture. Figure 13.3 shows a simple PCR setup that is used to amplify and visualize PCR products (amplicons).

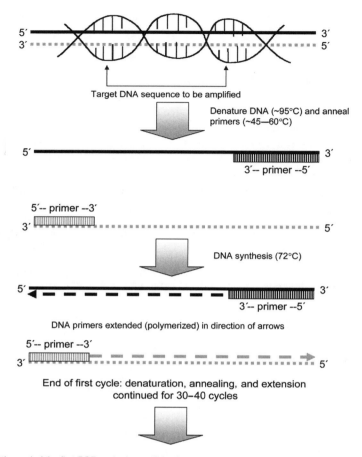

**Figure 13.2.** Schematic showing the PCR reaction, which is used to amplify specific DNA sequences.

**Table 13.2. Table showing the two common SNPs of 5,10MTHFR as examples to illustrate how the time-temperature coefficient for PCR cycling is varied very slightly to provide optimal amplicon synthesis. These conditions are used in the author's laboratory.**

| | | Stage 2 | | | | |
| | | 35 cycles of these three steps | | | | |
| | Stage 1 | Step 1 | Step 2 | Step 3 | Stage 3 | Hold amplicons at +4°C |
|---|---|---|---|---|---|---|
| **C677T MTHFR** | 95°C 2 mins | 95°C 60 s | 56°C 60 s | 72°C 60 s | 72°C 7 mins | 4°C |
| **A1298C MTHFR** | 95°C 5 mins, 55°C 2 mins, 72°C 2 mins | 95°C 75 s | 55°C 75 s | 72°C 90 s | 72°C 6 mins | 4°C |

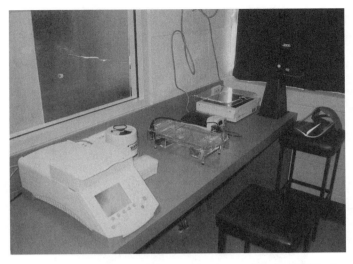

**Figure 13.3.** *A simple laboratory PCR setup based around the BioRad iCycler system.*

### 13.4.1   Restriction Enzyme Digestion of PCR Products to Detect SNPs

If the amplicon contains a base substitution that represents an important SNP (such as in the example of C677T-MTHFR), a restriction enzyme (bacterial endonuclease) can be used to digest the amplicon into oligonucleotide fragments, which differ according to whether they contain the base substitution. In the case of C677T-MTHFR, 0.5 $\mu$L of *Hinf*I (10 U/$\mu$L) is added for five hours at 37°C.

The fragments are then run on an electrophoresis system that contains ethidium bromide as a fluorescent DNA intercalating agent that permits band visualization under UV light. The pattern of bands allows for the determination of genotype. Figure 13.4 shows what banding pattern can be expected for the C677T-MTHFR SNP.

### 13.4.2   Real-Time PCR

Real-time PCR (RT–PCR) can be used to score SNPs without the need to use gels and dangerous chemicals such as ethidium bromide. It can also measure the number of copies of a gene or RNA molecule.

Instead of using a band in a gel as an endpoint, RT–PCR can measure the accumulation of an amplification product as the reaction progresses—hence "real time". To do this, the reaction mixture incorporates a fluorescent probe that reports an increase in DNA amplicon by a fluorescent signal that is directly proportional to the amount of DNA in the mixture.

If RT–PCR is used for genotyping (often referred to as allelic discrimination), it is common practice to use either TaqMan probes or Molecular Beacons. The TaqMan probes discriminate between allelic variants by using differentially labeled fluorescent probes that have allele specificity. That is, one probe is specific for the wildtype, and the other for the polymorphic allele. The probes are labeled differentially with a 5′ fluorescent reporter dye and a 3′ quencher. Fluorescence is only observed during the elongation phase of the PCR

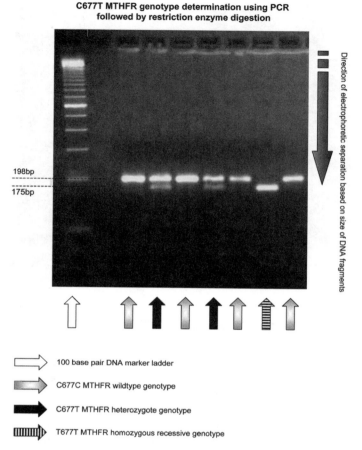

**Figure 13.4.** *After PCR amplification of a specific DNA sequence known to contain a gene polymorphism, restriction enzymes are used to digest the amplicon such that each genotype yields a different band pattern when polyacrylamide gel electrophoresis is performed. The figure shows the determination of C677T MTHFR genotype using this approach.*

cycle due to degradation by Taq-polymerase 5′ exonuclease activity, which separates the fluorophore from the quencher allowing a fluorescent signal to be emitted.

This signal is optimal for a perfectly matched probe compared with a mismatched probe whose signal remains quenched. It is this preferential hybridization that allows allelic discrimination and genotype scoring.

This kind of analysis can be multiplexed to permit rapid sample throughput for several SNP determinations.

## 13.5 PROTEIN MASS SPECTROMETRY

Two-dimensional polyacrylamide gel electrophoresis (2-D PAGE) separates a complex mixture of proteins according to both charge and mass. The stained protein "spots" are scanned to provide a signature that takes into account spatial and densitometric information. Differences in protein spot signature obtained under different sets of conditions or temporal profiles provide valuable information on differential protein expression that allows one to build up a "protein expression matrix."

Qualitative information on the nature of proteins visualized by 2D-PAGE can be augmented by applying matrix-assisted laser desorption/ionistion time-of-flight mass spectrometry (MALDI–TOF MS). Mass spectrometry is the accurate determination of the mass-charge ratio ($m/z$) of ions within a vacuum. This permits exact determination of molecular mass. MALDI–TOF MS is a relatively new technique that provides a powerful tool in modern protein biology. It can be used for large molecule analyses, including nucleic acid and protein sequencing, and ascertaining post-translational protein modifications. In the context of proteomics, it is perhaps best known for its ability to provide peptide-mass fingerprinting/fragment ion searching.

Peptide-mass fingerprinting involves enzyme cleavage (often a tryptic digest) and determination of resulting peptide masses using MALDI–TOF MS. The peptide fragment ions are correlated against a computer database to identify the original protein.

## 13.6 BIOINFORMATICS

Bioinformatics is a very new discipline within the life sciences. Modern biology generates a huge amount of information; just consider the output from measurements of gene expression experiments alone. For instance, the temporal changes in the transcriptome (RNA produced by our cells to adapt to changing conditions); post-transcriptional regulation; the variable expression matrix of translated proteins under the same changing conditions; the post-translational modifications to those proteins (i.e., phosphorylation, glycosylation, acetylation, demethylation, carboxylation, sulphation, and ubiquination) that influence activity. Add to this the outcome of modern techniques involving transgenics and RNA interference (iRNA), and you end up with more data than can be reasonably handled by any individual scientist, no matter what their intellect. To build up an idea of the interactome (Figure 1.10)—the ultimate in biological explanations of life processes—we need help.

Bioinformatics therefore brings together biology and information technology to cope with these large data sets. The world of bioinformatics involves the creation of databases for storage and interrogation. It permits for the comparison and statistical analysis between biological data in genomic and proteomic research. Essentially one can examine macro-molecular polymeric sequences (i.e., for DNA bases or protein amino acids), expression profiles, and three-dimensional structures.

In its simplest format, it allows scientists to interrogate scientific bibliographic databases to find relevant journal publications within a given field. Figure 13.5 shows a quick search for MTHFR in the NCBI PubMed site, which is a service of the National Library of Medicine and the National Institutes of Health http://www.ncbi.nlm.nih.gov/entrez/query.fcgi.

Other bibliographic databases also exist, for example, Scirus and Ovid:

http://www. scirus.com/srsapp/

http://www.ovid.com/site/index.jsp

Clearly, the Internet and advent of powerful personal computers for the masses has enabled bioinformatics to reach all interested scientists.

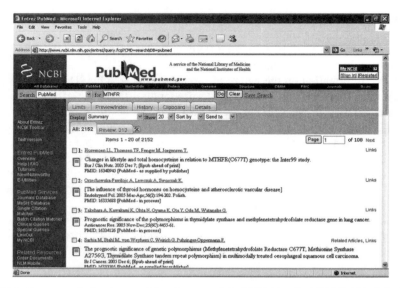

**Figure 13.5.** *Screen grab showing a quick online search for MTHFR in the NCBI PubMed site. This site is one of the best online resources for published journal articles.*

To search for DNA or protein sequence similarities, scientists generally resort to a basic local alignment search tool (BLAST) program. There are various examples available at the NCBI BLAST site. To illustrate how this works with a simple example, I performed a nucleotide–nucleotide BLAST (blastn) search in which I interrogated the database with the forward primer sequence of the common C677T-MTHFR SNP. The input interface is shown in Figure 13.6, whereas the output information, which clearly identifies 5,10MTHFR as the

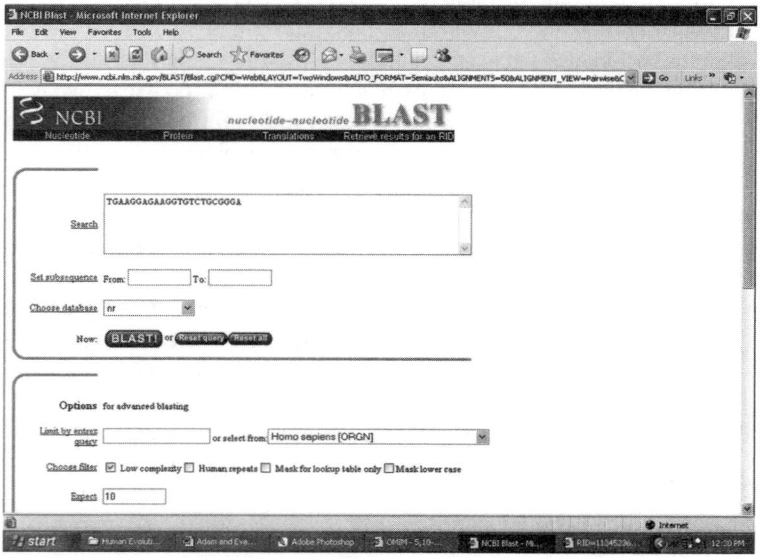

**Figure 13.6.** *Screen grab showing the nucleotide–nucleotide BLAST (blastn) interface with a query based on a partial (23 nucleotide) MTHFR sequence, which represents the forward primer used to detect C677T-MTFR.*

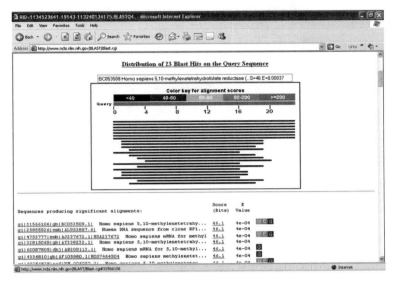

**Figure 13.7.** *Top genes that produce significant alignments for a blastn search based on a partial (23 nucleotide) MTHFR sequence that is represented by the C677T-MTHFR primer. Clearly, the database search has identified the correct gene.*

gene from which this sequence originates, is given in Figures 13.7 and 13.8. Figure 13.7 shows the top sequences that produce significant alignments, whereas Figure 13.8 shows the actual base alignment of the query (MTHFR primer) versus the database sequence for the two most significant alignments. The whole process took around 10 seconds.

Another useful site to find out information regarding specific genes is OMIM (online mendelian inheritance in man):

http://www.ncbi.nlm.nih.gov/entrez/dispomim.cgi?id= 607093

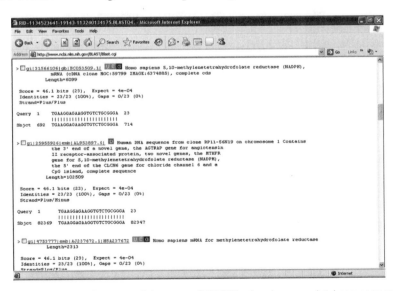

**Figure 13.8.** *Actual base alignment of the query (MTHFR primer) versus database sequence for the two most significant alignments.*

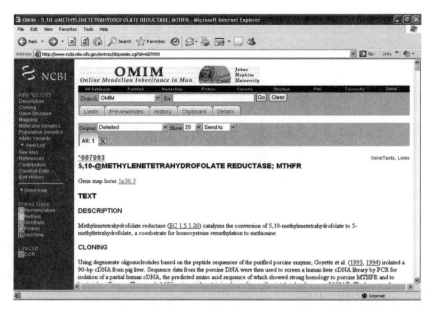

**Figure 13.9.** *A very useful site to find out information regarding specific genes is OMIM (online mendelian inheritance in man). The screen grab shows an OMIM search for MTHFR.*

Maintaining the theme of MTHFR, I have interrogated this site with this enzymes common acronym, and generated much information on the gene as shown in the screen grab given in Figure 13.9.

When you begin to use these kinds of database systems you will discover unique file formats such as NBRF/PIR and FASTA that provide a universal standard for bioinformatics data.

This fascinating area is set to expand and evolve over the coming years; already it has a range and depth that is well beyond the scope of this text. I will end by illustrating the need to create and interrogate such databases; just consider that the draft human genome project has already registered 1.4 million SNPs—that is 1 per 1000 to 2000 DNA bases. It is this circa 0.1% difference between any two individuals that contributes to humankind's genetic diversity and, hence, to our individuality.

# *References*

1. Gagneux P, Wills C, Gerloff U, Tautz D, Morin PA, Boesch C, Fruth B, Hohmann G, Ryder OA, Woodruff DS. Mitochondrial sequences show diverse evolutionary histories of African hominoids. Proc Natl Acad Sci U S A. 1999; 96: 5077–82.
2. Kaput J, Rodriguez RL. Nutritional genomics: the next frontier in the postgenomic era. Physiol Genomics. 2004; 16: 166–77.
3. Robinson GE, Grozinger CM, Whitfield CW. Sociogenomics: social life in molecular terms. Nat Rev Genet. 2005; 6: 257–70.
4. Rambaut A. Estimating the rate of molecular evolution: incorporating non-contemporaneous sequences into maximum likelihood phylogenies. Bioinformatics 2000; 16: 395–9.
5. Rambaut A, Bromham L. Estimating divergence dates from molecular sequences. Mol Biol Evol. 1998; 15: 442–48.
6. Bromham L, Penny D. The modern molecular clock. Nat Rev Genet. 2003; 4: 216–24.
7. Carroll SB. Genetics and the making of Homo sapiens. Nature. 2003; 422: 849–57.
8. Cantalupo C, Hopkins WD. Asymmetric Broca's area in great apes. Nature. 2001; 414: 505.
9. Gillies P. Nutrigenomics: the rubicon of molecular nutrition. Am Dietet Assoc. 2003; 103: S50–4.
10. Elliott R, Ong TJ. Nutritional genomics. BMJ. 2002; 324: 1438–42.
11. Ommen BV, Stierum R. Nutrigenomics: Exploiting systems biology in the nutrition and health arena. Curr Opin Biotechnol. 2002; 13: 517–21.
12. Milton K. Nutritional characteristics of wild primate foods: do the diets of our closest living relatives have lessons for us? Nutrition. 1999; 15: 488–98.
13. Aiello LC, Wheeler P. The expensive-tissue hypothesis. The brain and the digestive system in human and primate evolution. Curr Anthropol. 1995; 36: 199–221.
14. Dall SR, Boyd IL. Evolution of mammals: lactation helps mothers to cope with unreliable food supplies. Proc Biol Sci. 2004; 271: 2049–57.
15. Bayoumi RA, Flatz SD, Kuhnau W, Flatz G. Beja and Nilotes: nomadic pastoralist groups in the Sudan with opposite distributions of the adult lactase phenotypes. Am J Phys Anthropol. 1982; 58: 173–8.
16. Beja-Pereira A, Luikart G, England PR, Bradley DG, Jann OC, Bertorelle G, Chamberlain AT, Nunes TP, Metodiev S, Ferrand N, Erhardt G. Gene-culture coevolution between cattle milk protein genes and human lactase genes. Nat Genet. 2003; 35: 311–13.

17. Campbell AK, Matthews SB. Darwin's illness revealed. Postgrad Med J. 2005; 81: 248–51.

18. Loomis WF. Skin-pigment regulation of vitamin D biosynthjesis in man. Science. 1967; 157: 501–6.

19. Jablonski NG, Chaplin G. The evolution of skin color. J Hum Evol. 2000; 39: 57–106.

20. Lucock M, Yates Z, Glanville T, Leeming R, Simpson R, Daskalakis I. A critical role for B-vitamin nutrition in human developmental and evolutionary biology. Nutrition Res. 2003; 23: 1463–75.

21. Rees, JL. The genetics of sun sensitivity in humans. Am J Hum Genet. 2004: 75: 739–51.

22. Graf J, Hodgson R, van Daal A. Single nucleotide polymorphisms in the MATP gene are associated with normal human pigmentation variation. Hum Mutat. 2005; 25: 278–84.

23. Lucock M. Folic acid: nutritional biochemistry, molecular biology and role in disease processes. Molec Genet Metab 2000; 71: 121–38.

24. Lucock M, Ng X, Veysey M, Yates Z. Folic acid; an essential nutrient with added health benefits. Biologist. 2005; 52: 21–7.

25. Lucock M, Yates Z. Folic acid: Vitamin Panacea or Genetic Time Bomb. 'Perspectives – Opinion' Nat Rev Genet. 2005; 6: 235–40.

26. Blau N, Bonafe L, Thony B. Tetrahydrobiopterin deficiencies without hyperphenylalaninemia: diagnosis and genetics of dopa-responsive dystonia and sepiapterin reductase deficiency. Mol Genet Metab 2001; 74: 172–85.

27. Moat SJ, Lang D, McDowell IF, Clarke ZL, Madhavan AK, Lewis MJ, Goodfellow J. Folate, homocysteine, endothelial function and cardiovascular disease. J Nutr Biochem. 2004; 15: 64–79.

28. Hayden MR, Tyagi SC. Homocysteine and reactive oxygen species in metabolic syndrome, type 2 diabetes mellitus, and atheroscleropathy: the pleiotropic effects of folate supplementation. Nutr J. 2004; 3: 4.

29. Stroes ES, van Faassen EE, Yo M, Martasek P, Boer P, Govers R, Rabelink TJ. Folic acid reverts dysfunction of endothelial nitric oxide synthase. Circ Res. 2000; 86: 1129–34.

30. Hyndman ME, Verma S, Rosenfeld RJ, Anderson TJ, Parsons HG. Am J Physiol Heart Circ Physiol. 2002; 282: 2167–72.

31. Blount JD. Carotenoids and life-history evolution in animals. Arch Biochem Biophys. 2004; 430: 10–5.

32. Wong WY, Merkus HM, Thomas CM, Menkveld R, Zielhuis GA, Steegers-Theunissen RP. Effects of folic acid and zinc sulfate on male factor subfertility: a double-blind, randomized, placebo-controlled trial. Fertil Steril. 2002; 77: 491–8.

33. Hansen JC, Deguchi Y. Selenium and fertility in animals and man–a review. Acta Vet Scand. 1996; 37: 19–30.

34. Xu DX, Shen HM, Zhu QX, Chua L, Wang QN, Chia SE, Ong CN. The associations among semen quality, oxidative DNA damage in human spermatozoa and concentrations of cadmium, lead and selenium in seminal plasma. Mutat Res. 2003; 534: 155–63.

35. Bedwal RS, Bahuguna A. Zinc, copper and selenium in reproduction. Experientia. 1994; 50: 626–40.

36. Hatfield DL, Gladyshev VN. How selenium has altered our understanding of the genetic code. Mol Cell Biol. 2002; 22: 3565–76.

37. Reyes-Engel A, Munoz E, Gaitan MJ, et al. Implications on human fertility of the 677C–>T and 1298A→C polymorphisms of the MTHFR gene: consequences of a possible genetic selection. Mol Hum Reprod 2002; 8: 952–7.

38. Green JM, Mackenzie RE, Matthews RG. Substrate flux through methylenetetrahydrofolate dehydrogenase: predicted effects of the concentration of methylenetetrahydrofolate on its partitioning into pathways leading to nucleotide biosynthesis or methionine regeneration. Biochem. 1988; 27: 8014–22.

39. Duthie SJ, Hawdon A. DNA instability (strand breakage, uracil misincorporation, and defective repair) is increased by folic acid depletion in human lymphocytes *in vitro*. FASEB J. 1998; 12: 1491–97.

40. Gu L, Wu J, Qiu L, Jennings CD, Li GM. Involvement of DNA mismatch repair in folate deficiency-induced apoptosis. J Nutr Biochem. 2002; 13: 355–63.

41. Isotalo PA, Wells GA, Donnelly JG. Neonatal and fetal methylenetetrahydrofolate reductase genetic polymorphisms: an examination of C677T and A1298C mutations. Am J Hum Genet. 2000; 67: 986–90.

42. Munoz-Moran E, Dieguez-Lucena JL, Fernandez-Arcas N, Peran-Mesa S, Reyes-Engel A. Genetic selection and folate intake during pregnancy. Lancet. 1998; 352: 1120–21.

43. Guenther BD, Sheppard CA, Tran P, Rozen R, Matthews RG, Ludwig M. The structure and properties of methylenetetrahydrofolate reductase from E. coli suggest how folate ameliorates human hyperhomocysteinemia. Nat Struct Biol. 1999; 6: 359–65.

44. Scholl TO, Hediger ML, Fischer RL, Shearer JW. Anemia vs iron deficiency: increased risk of preterm delivery in a prospective study. Am J Clin Nutr. 1992; 55: 985–8.

45. Merryweather-Clarke AT, Pointon JJ, Shearman JD, Robson KJ. Global prevalence of putative haemochromatosis mutations. J Med Genet. 1997; 34: 275–8.

46. Ajioka RS, Jorde LB, Gruen JR, Yu P, Dimitrova D, Barrow J, Radisky E, Edwards CQ, Griffen LM, Kushner JP. Haplotype analysis of hemochromatosis: evaluation of different linkage-disequilibrium approaches and evolution of disease chromosomes. Am J Hum Genet. 1997; 60: 1439–47.

47. Thomas W, Fullan A, Loeb DB, McClelland EE, Bacon BR, Wolff RK. A haplotype and linkage disequilibrium analysis of the hereditary hemochromatosis gene region. Hum Genet. 1998; 102: 5171–25.

48. Bulaj ZJ, Griffen LM, Jorde LB, Edwards CQ, Kushner JP. Clinical and biochemical abnormalities in people heterozygous for hemochromatosis. N Engl J Med. 1996; 335: 1799–805.

49. Lee KH, Choi E, Chun YS, Kim MS, Park JW. Differential responses of two degradation domains of HIF-1alpha to hypoxia and iron deficiency. Biochimie. 2006; 88: 163–9.

50. Luttun A, Carmeliet P. Soluble VEGF receptor Flt1: the elusive preeclampsia factor discovered? J Clin Invest. 2003; 111: 600–2.

51. Liu E, Percy MJ, Amos CI, Guan Y, Shete S, Stockton DW, McMullin MF, Polyakova LA, Ang SO, Pastore YD, Jedlickova K, Lappin TR, Gordeuk V, Prchal JT. The worldwide distribution of the VHL 598C>T mutation indicates a single founding event. Blood. 2004; 103: 1937–40.

52. Danpure CJ. Variable peroxisomal and mitochondrial targeting of alanine: glyoxylate aminotransferase in mammalian evolution and disease. Bioessays. 1997; 19: 317–26.

53. Caldwell EF, Mayor LR, Thomas MG, Danpure CJ. Diet and the frequency of the alanine: glyoxylate aminotransferase Pro11Leu polymorphism in different human populations. Hum Genet. 2004; 115: 504–9.

54. Lucock, M. Is folic acid the ultimate functional food component for disease prevention? Br Med J. 2004; 328: 211–14.

55. Isotalo PA, Wells GA, & Donnelly JG. Neonatal and fetal methylenetetrahydrofolate reductase genetic polymorphisms: an examination of C677T and A1298C mutations. Am J Hum Genet. 2000; 67: 986–90.

56. Duthie SJ, Hawdon A. DNA instability (strand breakage, uracil misincorporation, and defective repair) is increased by folic acid depletion in human lymphocytes in vitro. FASEB J. 1998; 12: 1491–97.

57. Eskes TK. Homocysteine and human reproduction. Clin Exp Obstet Gynecol. 2000; 27: 157–67.

58. van Aerts LAGJM. Embryotoxicity studies on cyclophosphamide and homocysteine. Thesis Katholieke Universiteit Nijmegen. 1995.

59. Corbo RM, Scacchi R. Apolipoprotein E (APOE) allele distribution in the world. Is APOE*4 a 'thrifty' allele? Ann Hum Genet. 1999; 63: 301–10.

60. Corbo RM, Scacchi R, Cresta M. Differential reproductive efficiency associated with common apolipoprotein e alleles in postreproductive-aged subjects. Fertil Steril. 2004; 81: 104–7.

61. Jenkins DJ, Kendall CW, Marchie A, Jenkins AL, Connelly PW, Jones PJ, Vuksan V. The Garden of Eden–plant based diets, the genetic drive to conserve cholesterol and its implications

for heart disease in the 21st century. Comp Biochem Physiol A Mol Integr Physiol. 2003; 136: 141–51.

62. Ordovas JM, Cupples LA, Corella D, Otvos JD, Osgood D, Martinez A, Lahoz C, Coltell O, Wilson PW, Schaefer EJ. Association of cholesteryl ester transfer protein-TaqIB polymorphism with variations in lipoprotein subclasses and coronary heart disease risk: the Framingham study. Arterioscler Thromb Vasc Biol. 2000; 20: 1323–9.

63. Galluzzi JR, Cupples LA, Otvos JD, Wilson PW, Schaefer EJ, Ordovas JM. Association of the A/T54 polymorphism in the intestinal fatty acid binding protein with variations in plasma lipids in the Framingham Offspring Study. Atherosclerosis. 2001; 159: 417–24.

64. Lev-Ran A, Porta M. Salt and hypertension: a phylogenetic perspective. Diabetes Met Res Rev. 2005; 21: 118–31.

65. Poch E, Gonzalez D, Giner V, Bragulat E, Coca A, de La Sierra A. Molecular basis of salt sensitivity in human hypertension. Evaluation of renin-angiotensin-aldosterone system gene polymorphisms. Hypertension. 2001; 38: 1204–9.

66. Danziger RS. Hypertension in an anthropological and evolutionary paradigm. Hypertension. 2001; 38: 19–22.

67. Wilson TW, Grim CE. Biohistory of slavery and blood pressure differences in blacks today. A hypothesis. Hypertension. 1991; 17(Suppl. 1): 122–28.

68. Weinberger MH. Salt sensitivity of blood pressure in humans. Hypertension. 1996; 27: 481–90.

69. Curtin PD. The slavery hypothesis for hypertension among African Americans: the historical evidence. Am J Public Health. 1992; 82: 1681–6.

70. Ruiz-Narvaez E. Is the Ala12 variant of the PPARG gene an "unthrifty allele". J Med Genet. 2005; 42: 547–50.

71. Auwerx J. PPARgamma, the ultimate thrifty gene. Diabetologia. 1999; 42: 1033–49.

72. Deeb SS, Fajas L, Nemoto M, Pihlajamaki J, Mykkanen L, Kuusisto J, Laakso M, Fujimoto W, Auwerx J. A Pro12Ala substitution in PPARgamma2 associated with decreased receptor activity, lower body mass index and improved insulin sensitivity. Nat Genet. 1998; 20: 284–7.

73. Drewnowski A, Gomez-Carneros C. Bitter taste, phytonutrients, and the consumer: a review. Am J Clin Nutr. 2000; 72: 1424–35.

74. Soranzo N, Bufe B, Sabeti PC, Wilson JF, Weale ME, Marguerie R, Meyerhof W, Goldstein DB. Positive selection on a high-sensitivity allele of the human bitter-taste receptor TAS2R16. Curr Biol. 2005; 15: 1257–65.

75. Chandrashekar J, Mueller KL, Hoon MA, Adler E, Feng L, Guo W, Zuker CS, Ryba NJ. T2Rs function as bitter taste receptors. Cell. 2000; 100: 703–11.

76. Osier MV, Pakstis AJ, Soodyall H, Comas D, Goldman D, Odunsi A, Okonofua F, Parnas J, Schulz LO, Bertranpetit J, Bonne-Tamir B, Lu RB, Kidd JR, Kidd KK. A global perspective on genetic variation at the ADH genes reveals unusual patterns of linkage disequilibrium and diversity. Am J Hum Genet. 2002; 71: 84–99.

77. Lang M, Pelkonen O. Metabolism of xenobiotics and chemical carcinogenesis. IARC Sci Publ. 1999; 148: 13–22.

78. Ingelman-Sundberg M. The human genome project and novel aspects of cytochrome P450 research. Toxicol Appl Pharmacol. 2005; 207: 52–6.

79. Ames BN. DNA damage from micronutrient deficiencies is likely to be a major cause of cancer. Mut Res. 2001; 475: 7–20.

80. Langlois MR, Delanghe JR, De Buyzere ML, Bernard DR, Ouyang J. Effect of haptoglobin on the metabolism of vitamin C. Am J Clin Nutr. 1997; 66: 606–10.

81. Langlois MR, Delanghe JR. Biological and clinical significance of haptoglobin polymorphism in humans. Clin Chem. 1996; 42: 1589–600.

82. Azzi A, Gysin R, Kempna P, Munteanu A, Negis Y, Villacorta L, Visarius T, Zingg JM. Vitamin E mediates cell signaling and regulation of gene expression. Ann N Y Acad Sci. 2004; 1031: 86–95.

83. Guy, M. Vitamin D receptor gene polymorphisms and breast cancer risk. Clin Cancer Res. 2004; 10: 5472–81.

84. Walsh CT, Sandstead HH, Prasad AS, Newberne PM, Fraker PJ. Zinc: health effects and research priorities for the 1990s. Environ Health Perspect. 1994; 102: 5–46.

85. Oteiza PI, Olin KL, Fraga CG, Keen CL. Zinc deficiency causes oxidative damage to proteins, lipids and DNA in rat testes. J Nutr. 1995; 125: 823–9.

86. Halliwell B, Gutteridge JMC. Free Radicals in Biology and Medicine. 1999; Clarendon Press, Oxford.

87. Strain JJ, Benzie IFF. Antioxidants: diet and antioxidant defence. 1999; In: Sadler M, Strain JJ, Cabellero B (eds) The Encyclopedia of Human Nutrition. Academic Press, London, pp 95–106.

88. Ochiai EI. Copper and the biological evolution. BioSystems. 1983; 16: 81–6.

89. Shayeghi M, Latunde-Dada GO, Oakhill JS, Laftah AH, Takeuchi K, Halliday N, Khan Y, Warley A, McCann FE, Hider RC, Frazer DM, Anderson GJ, Vulpe CD, Simpson RJ, McKie AT. Identification of an intestinal heme transporter. Cell. 2005; 122: 789–801.

90. Fukuhara R, Tezuka T, Kageyama T. Structure, molecular evolution, and gene expression of primate superoxide dismutases. Gene. 2002; 296: 99–109.

91. Mann N. Dietary lean red meat and human evolution. Eur J Nutr. 2000; 39: 71–9.

92. Crawford M. The role of dietary fatty acids in biology: their place in the evolution of the human brain. Nutr Rev. 1992; 50: 3–11.

93. Chamberlain JG. The possible role of long-chain omega–3 fatty acids in human brain phylogeny. Persp Biol Med. 1996; 39: 436–445.

94. Martin RD. Relative brain size and metabolic rate in terrestrial vertebrates. Nature. 1981; 293: 57–60.

95. Mann FD. Animal fat and cholesterol may have helped primitive man evolve a large brain. Persp Biol Med. 1998; 41: 417–425.

96. Crawford MA. The role of dietary fatty acids in biology: their place in the evolution of the human brain. Nutr Rev. 1992; 50: 3–11.

97. Aiello LC, Wheeler P. The expensive tissue hypothesis. Curr Anthropology. 1995; 36: 199–332.

98. Erren TC, Erren M. Can fat explain the human brain's big bang evolution?-Horrobin's leads for comparative and functional genomics. Prostaglandins Leukot Essent Fatty Acids. 2004; 70: 345–7.

99. Evans PD, Anderson JR, Vallender EJ, Gilbert SL, Malcom CM, Dorus S, Lahn BT. Adaptive evolution of ASPM, a major determinant of cerebral cortical size in humans. Hum Mol Genet. 2004; 13: 489–94.

100. Kouprina N, Pavlicek A, Mochida GH, Solomon G, Gersch W, Yoon YH, Collura R, Ruvolo M, Barrett JC, Woods CG, Walsh CA, Jurka J, Larionov V. Accelerated evolution of the ASPM gene controlling brain size begins prior to human brain expansion. PLoS Biol. 2004; 2: E126.

101. Correia HR, Balseiro SC, de Areia ML. Are genes of human intelligence related to the metabolism of thyroid and steroids hormones?—endocrine changes may explain human evolution and higher intelligence. Med Hypotheses. 2005; 65: 1016–23.

102. Gilbert SL, Dobyns WB, Lahn BT. Genetic links between brain development and brain evolution. Nat Rev Genet. 2005; 6: 581–90.

103. Kennedy GE. From the ape's dilemma to the weanling's dilemma: early weaning and its evolutionary context. J Hum Evol. 2005; 48: 123–45.

104. Turner AJ. The relationship between brain folate and monoamine metabolism. 1979; In: Botez MI, Reynolds EH (ed) Folic Acid in Neurology, Psychiatry, and Internal Medicine. Raven Press, New York, pp 165–177.

105. Godfrey PSA, Toone BK, Carney MWP, Flynn T, Bottiglieri T, Laudy M, Chanarin I, Reynolds E. Enhancement of recovery from psychiatric illness by methylfolate. Lancet. 1990; 336: 392–5.

106. Hamer DH. The god gene: how faith is hardwired into our genes. 2004; Doubleday, New York.

107. Lorenzi C, Serretti A, Mandelli L, Tubazio V, Ploia C, Smeraldi E. 5-HT(1A) polymorphism and self-transcendence in mood disorders. Am J Med Genet Part B (Neuropsychiatr Genet). 2005; 137: 33–5.

108. Shank RP, Aprison MH. The metabolism in vivo of glycine and serine in eight areas of the rat central nervous system. J Neurochem. 1970; 17: 1461–75.

109. Bourne MG, Sharma SK, Spector RG. The effects of folate on neurotransmitter uptake into rat cerebral cortex slices. Biochem Pharmacol. 1976; 25: 1917–8.

110. Lucock MD, Green M, Levene MI. Methylfolate modulates potassium evoked neuro-secretion: evidence for a role at the pteridine cofactor level of tyrosine 3-hydroxylase. Neurochem Res. 1995; 20: 727–36.

111. Lucock M, Yates Z, Hall K, Leeming R, Rylance G, MacDonald A, Green A. The impact of phenylketonuria on folate metabolism. Mol Genet Metab. 2002; 76: 305–12.

112. Lucock MD, Levene MI, Hartley R. Modulation of potassium evoked secretory function in rat cerebellar slices measured by real time monitoring: evidence of a possible role for methylfolate in cerebral tissue. Neurochem Res. 1993; 18: 617–23.

113. Olney JW, Fuller TA, de Gubareff T. Kainate-like neurotoxicity of folates. Nature. 1981; 292: 165–7.

114. Borg J, Andree B, Soderstrom H, Farde L. The serotonin system and spiritual experiences. Am J Psychiatry. 2003; 160: 1965–9.

115. Caporael LR. Ergotism: the satan loosed in Salem? Science. 1976; 192: 21–6.

116. Graham JB, Dudley R, Aguilar AM, Gans C. Implication of the late palaeozoic oxygen pulse for physiology and evolution. Nature. 1995: 375: 117–20.

117. Benzie IF. Evolution of dietary antioxidants. Comp Biochem Physiol A Mol Integr Physiol. 2003; 136: 113–26.

118. Chatterjee IB. Evolution and biosynthesis of ascorbic acid. Science. 1973; 182: 1271–2.

119. Pauling L. Evolution and the need for ascorbic acid. Proc Natl Acad Sci. 1970; 67:1643–8.

120. Nandi A, Mukhopadhyay CK, Ghosh MK, Chattopadhyay DJ, Chatterjee IB. Evolutionary significance of vitamin C biosynthesis in terrestrial vertebrates. Free Rad Biol Med. 1997; 22: 1047–54.

121. Millar J. Vitamin C – the primate fertility factor? Med Hypotheses.1992; 38: 292–5.

122. Calabrese EJ. Evolutionary loss of ascorbic acid synthesis: how it may have enhanced the survival interests of man. Med Hypotheses. 1982; 8: 173–5.

123. Challem JJ. Did the loss of endogenous ascorbate propel the evolution of Anthropoidea and Homo sapiens? Med Hypotheses. 1997; 48: 387–92.

124. Banhegyi G, Braun L, Csala M, Puska F, Mandl J. Ascorbate metabolism and its regulation in animals. Free Rad Biol Med. 1997; 23: 793–803.

125. Cutler RG. Antioxidants and aging. Am J Clin Nutr. 1991; 53: S373–9.

126. Ames BN, Cathcart R, Schwiers E, Hochstein P. Uric acid provides an antioxidant defense in humans against oxidant- and radical-caused aging and cancer: a hypothesis. Proc Natl Acad Sci. 1981; 78: 6858–62.

127. Fridovich I. Superoxide anion radical, superoxide dismutases and related matters. J Biol Chem. 1997; 272: 18515–7.

128. Fridovich I. Oxygen toxicity: a radical explanation. J Exp Biol. 1998; 210: 1203–9.

129. Barja G. Oxygen radicals, a failure or a success of evolution? Free Rad Res Comm. 1993; 18: 63–70.

130. Jackson MJ, McArdle A, McArdle F. Antioxidant micronutrients and gene expression. Proc Nutr Soc. 1998; 57: 310–5.

131. Haig D. Evolutionary conflicts in pregnancy and calcium metabolism. Placenta. 2004; 25: Supp A Troph Res. 18: S10–5.

132. Levitan RD, Masellis M, Lam RW, Kaplan AS, Davis C, Tharmalingam S, Mackenzie B, Basile VS, Kennedy JL. A birth-season/DRD4 gene interaction predicts weight gain and obesity in

women with seasonal affective disorder: A seasonal thrifty phenotype hypothesis. Neuropsy-chopharmacology. In Press.

133. Paoloni-Giacobino A. A conflict within the genome, the battle of the sexes? Rev Med Suisse. 2005; 1: 1687–90.

134. Boyd R, Silk JB. How Humans Evolved. 2000; W.W.Norton & Company. New York.

135. Illius AW, Tolkamp BJ, Yearsley J. The evolution of the control of food intake. Proc Nutr Soc. 2002; 61: 465–72.

136. Parkes TL, Elia AJ, Dickinson D, Hilliker AJ, Phillips JP, Boulianne GL. Extension of Drosophila lifespan by overexpression of human SOD1 in motorneurons. Nat Genet. 1998; 19: 171–4.

137. Strassman B. Energy economy in the evolution of menstruation. Evolutionary Anthropology. 1996; 5: 157–64.

138. Walker R, Hill K. Modeling growth and senescence in physical performance among the Ache of Eastern Paraguay. Am J Hum Biol. 2003; 15: 196–208.

139. Blurton Jones NG, Hawkes K, O'Connell JF. Antiquity of postreproductive life: are there modern impacts on hunter-gatherer postreproductive life spans? Am J Hum Biol. 2002; 14:184–205.

140. Caspari R, Lee S-H. Older age becomes common in human evolution. Proc Natl Acad Sci. 2004; 10: 10895–900.

141. Stewart CB, Wilson AC. Sequence convergence and functional adaptation of stomach lysozymes from foregut fermenters. Cold Spring Harb Symp Quant Biol. 1987; 52: 891–9.

142. Eaton SB, Eaton SB 3rd, Konner MJ. Paleolithic nutrition revisited: a twelve-year retrospective on its nature and implications. Eur J Clin Nutr. 1997; 51: 207–16.

143. Eaton SB, Strassman BI, Nesse RM, Neel JV, Ewald PW, Williams GC, Weder AB, Eaton SB 3rd, Lindeberg S, Konner MJ, Mysterud I, Cordain L. Evolutionary health promotion. Prev Med. 2002; 34: 109–18.

144. Tattersall I. Becoming human. Evolution and human uniqueness. 1998, Harcourt Brace, New York, p 239.

145. Johanson D. Reading the minds of fossils. Sci Am. 1998; 278: 102–3.

146. Rendine S, Piazza A, Cavalli-Sforza LL. Simulation and separation by principle components of multiple demic expansions in Europe. Am Nat. 1986; 128: 681–706.

147. Cavalli-Sforza LL, Menozzi P, Piazza A. Demic expansions and human evolution. Science. 1993; 259: 639–46.

148. Eades MK, Eades MD. Protein Power. 1996; Bantam Press, New York.

149. McCully KS. The significance of wheat in the Dakota Territory, human evolution, civilization, and degenerative diseases. Perspect Biol Med. 2001; 44: 52–61.

150. Cleave TL. The saccharine disease. 1974; Wright, Bristol.

151. McCully K S, McCully ME. The heart revolution. 1999; Harper-Collins, New York.

152. Carson NAJ, Neill DW. Metabolic abnormalities detected in a survey of mentally backward individuals in Northern Ireland. Arch Dis Child. 1962; 37: 505–13.

153. Mudd SH, Finkelstein JD, Irreverre F, Laster L. Homocystinuria: an enzymatic defect. Science. 1964; 143: 1443–5.

154. Mudd SH, Levy HL, Skovby F. Disorders of transsulfuration. In: Scriver CR, Beaudet AL, Sly WS, Walle D (eds) The Metabolic and Molecular Basis of Inherited Disease. 1995; McGrawHill, New York, pp 1279–338.

155. Harker LA, Slichter SJ, Scott CR, Ross R. Homocystinemia vascular injury and arterial throm-bosis. N Engl J Med 1974; 291: 537–43.

156. Ueland PM, Refsum H, Brattstrom L. Plasma homocysteine and cardiovascular disease. In: Francis RB Jr (ed) Atherosclerotic cardiovascular disease, hemostasis, and endothelial function. 1992; Marcel Dekker, NewYork, pp 183–236.

157. Stampfer MJ, Malinow MR. Can lowering homocystine levels reduce cardiovascular risk. New Eng J Med. 1995; 332: 328–9.

158. Motulsky AG. Nutritional ecogenetics: Homocysteine related arteriosclerotic vascular disease, neural tube defects and folic acid. Am J Hum Genet. 1996; 58: 17–20.

159. Verhoeff P, Stampfer MJ. Prospective studies of homocysteine and cardiovascular disease. Nutr Rev. 1995; 33: 283–8.
160. Alfthan G, Pakkanen J, Jaubirmen M. Relation of serum homocysteine and lipoprotein (A) concentrations to atherosclerotic disease in a prospective Finnish population based study. Atherosclerosis. 1994; 106: 9–16.
161. Perry IJ, Refsum H, Morris RW, Ebrabim SB, Ueland PM, Shaper AC. Prospective study of serum total homocysteine concentrations and risk of stroke in middle aged British men. Lancet. 1995; 346: 1395–8.
162. Petri M, Roubenhoff R, Dallal GE, Nadeau MR, Selhub J, Rosenberg IH. Plasma homocysteine as a risk factor for atherothrombotic events in systematic lupus erythematosus. Lancet. 1996; 348: 1120–24.
163. Malinow MR, Nieto FJ, Szklo M, Chambless LE, Bond G. Carotid artery intimal-medial thickening and plasma homocysteine in asymptomatic adults: the atherosclerosis risk in communities study. Circulation. 1993; 87: 1107–13.
164. Selhub J, Jacques PF, Boston AG. Association between plasma homocysteine concentration and extracranial carotid-artery stenosis. N Engl J Med. 1995; 332: 286–91.
165. Frosst P, Blom HJ, Milos R, Goyette P, Sheppard CA, Matthews RG, Boers GJ, den Heijer M, Kluijtmans LA, Van den Heuvel LP. A candidate genetic risk factor for vascular disease: a common mutation in methylenetetrahydrofolate reductase. Nat Genet. 1995; 10: 111–3.
166. Flegal KM, Carroll MD, Ogden CL, Johnson C L. Prevalence and trends in obesity among US adults, 1999–2000. JAMA. 2002; 288: 1723–7.
167. French SA, Story M, Jeffery RW. Environmental influences on eating and physical activity. Annu Rev Public Health. 2001; 22: 309–35.
168. Bell CG, Walley AJ, Froguel P. The genetics of human obesity. Nat Rev Genet. 2005; 6: 221–34.
169. Neel JV. Diabetes mellitus: a 'thrifty' genotype rendered detrimental by 'progress'? Am J Hum Genet. 1962; 14: 353–62.
170. Friedman JM. A war on obesity, not the obese. Science. 2003; 299: 856–8.
171. Cossrow N, Falkner B. Race/ethnic issues in obesity and obesity-related comorbidities. J Clin Endocrinol Metab. 2004; 89: 2590–4.
172. Brookfield JFY. Human evolution: A legacy of cannibalism in our genes? Curr Biol. 2003; 13: R592–3.
173. Mead S, Stumpf MP, Whitfield J, Beck JA, Poulter M, Campbell T, Uphill JB, Goldstein D, Alpers M, Fisher EM, Collinge J. Balancing selection at the prion protein gene consistent with prehistoric kurulike epidemics. Science. 2003; 300: 640–3.
174. Willett WC, Sacks F, Trichopoulou A. Mediterranean diet pyramid: a cultural model for healthy eating. Am J Clin Nutr. 1995; 61: S1402–6.
175. Visioli F, Grande S, Bogani P, Galli C. The role of antioxidants in the Mediterranean diets: focus on cancer. Eur J Cancer Prev 2004; 13: 337–43.
176. Trichopoulou A, Critselis E. Mediterranean diet and longevity. Eur J Cancer Prev. 2004; 13: 453–56.
177. Hasler CM. Functional foods: benefits, concerns and challenges-a position paper from the American Council on Science and Health. J Nutr. 2002; 132: 3772–81.
178. Christen WG, Buring JE, Manson JE, Hennekens CH. Beta-carotene supplementation: a good thing, a bad thing, or nothing? Curr Opin Lipidol. 1999; 10: 29–33.
179. The Alpha-Tocopherol Beta Carotene Cancer Prevention Study Group. The effect of vitamin E and beta carotene on the incidence of lung cancer and other cancers in male smokers. N Engl J Med. 1994; 330: 1029–35.
180. Omenn GS, Goodman GE, Thornquist MD. Effects of a combination of beta carotene and vitamin A on lung cancer and cardiovascular disease. N Engl J Med. 1996; 334: 1150–55.
181. Visioli F, Bogani P, Grande S, Galli C. Mediterranean food and health: building human evidence. J Physiol Pharmacol. 2005; 56 Suppl. 1: 37–49.

182. Visioli F, Riso P, Grande S, Galli C, Porrini M. Protective activity of tomato products on in vivo markers of lipid oxidation. Eur J Nutr. 2003; 42: 201–6.

183. Murphy KJ, Chronopoulos AK, Singh I, Francis MA, Moriarty H, Pike MJ, Turner AH, Mann NJ, Sinclair AJ. Dietary flavanols and procyanidin oligomers from cocoa (Theobroma cacao) inhibit platelet function. Am J Clin Nutr. 2003; 77: 1466–73.

184. Tyagi A, Agarwal R, Agarwal C. Grape seed extract inhibits EGF-induced and constitutively active mitogenic signaling but activates JNK in human prostate carcinoma DU145 cells: possible role in antiproliferation and apoptosis. Oncogene. 2003; 22: 1302–16.

185. Ye X, Krohn RL, Liu W, Joshi SS, Kuszynski CA, McGinn TR, Bagchi M, Preuss HG, Stohs SJ, Bagchi D. The cytotoxic effects of a novel IH636 grape seed proanthocyanidin extract on cultured human cancer cells. Mol Cell Biochem. 1999; 196: 99–108.

186. Muskiet FA, Fokkema MR, Schaafsma A, Boersma ER, Crawford MA. Is docosahexaenoic acid (DHA) essential? Lessons from DHA status regulation, our ancient diet, epidemiology and randomized controlled trials. J Nutr. 2004; 134: 183–6.

187. Simopoulos AP. Essential fatty acids in health and chronic disease. Am J Clin Nutr. 1999; 70: S560–9.

188. Price PT, Nelson CM, Clarke SD. Omega-3 polyunsaturated fatty acid regulation of gene expression. Curr Opin Lipidol. 2000; 11: 3–7.

189. Horton JD, Shimomura I. Sterol regulatory element-binding proteins: activators of cholesterol and fatty acid biosynthesis. Curr Opin Lipidol. 1999; 10: 143–50.

190. Innis SM. Essential fatty acids in growth and development. Prog Lipid Res. 1991; 30: 39–103.

191. Burdge GC, Jones AE, Wootton SA. Eicosapentaenoic and docosapentaenoic acids are the principal products of alpha-linolenic acid metabolism in young men. Br J Nutr. 2002; 88: 355–63.

192. Smit EN, Fokkema MR, Boersma ER, Muskiet FA. Higher erythrocyte 22:6n-3 and 22:5n-6, and lower 22:5n-3 suggest higher delta-4-desaturation capacity in women of childbearing age. Br J Nutr. 2003; 89: 739–40.

193. Burdge GC, Wootton SA. Conversion of alpha-linolenic acid to eicosapentaenoic, docosapentaenoic and docosahexaenoic acids in young women. Br J Nutr. 2002; 88: 411–20.

194. Forsyth JS, Carlson SE. Long-chain polyunsaturated fatty acids in infant nutrition: effects on infant development. Curr Opin Clin Nutr Metab Care. 2001; 4: 123–6.

195. Makrides M, Neumann MA, Jeffrey B, Lien EL, Gibson R A. A randomized trial of different ratios of linoleic to alpha-linolenic acid in the diet of term infants: effects on visual function and growth. Am J Clin Nutr. 2000; 71: 120–9.

196. Gibbons A. American Association of Physical Anthropologists meeting. Humans' head start: new views of brain evolution. Science. 2002; 296: 835–7.

197. Broadhurst CL, Wang Y, Crawford MA, Cunnane SC, Parkington JE Schmidt WF. Brain-specific lipids from marine, lacustrine, or terrestrial food resources: potential impact on early African Homo sapiens. Comp Biochem Physiol B Biochem. Mol Biol 2002; 131: 653–73.

198. Muller M, Kersten S. Nutrigenomics: goals and strategies. Nature Rev Genet. 2003; 4: 315–22.

199. Lucock M, Yates Z. Synergy between *677 TT* MTHFR genotype and related folate SNPs regulates homocysteine level. Nutrition Research. 2006; 26: 180–5.

200. Matthews RG, Cobalamin-dependent methyltransferases, Acc Chem Res. 2001; 34: 681–9.

201. Oteanu H, Banerjee R, Human methionine synthase reductase, a soluble P 450 reductase-like dual flavoprotein, is sufficient for NADPH-dependent methionine synthase activation, J Biol Chem. 2001; 276: 35558–63.

202. Dufficy L, Naumovski N, Ng X, Blades B, Yates Z, Travers C, Lewis P, Sturm J, Veysey M, Roach P, Lucock M. G80A reduced folate carrier SNP influences the absorption and cellular translocation of dietary folate and its association with blood pressure in an elderly population. Life Sciences; 2006; 79: 957–66.

203. Nguye TT, Dyer DL, Dunning DD, Rubin SA, Grant KE, Said HM. Human intestinal folate transport: cloning, expression, and distribution of complementary RNA. Gastroenterology. 1997; 112: 783–91.

204. Prasad PD, Ramamoorthy S, Leibach FH, Ganapathy V. Molecular cloning of the human placental folate transporter. Biochem Biophys Res Comm. 1995; 206: 681–7.

205. Moscow JA, Gong M., He R, Sgagias MK, Dixon KH, Anzick SL, Meltzer PS, Cowan KH. Isolation of a gene encoding a human reduced folate carrier (RFC1) and analysis of its expression in transport-deficient, methotrexate-resistant human breast cancer cells. Cancer Research. 1995; 55: 3790–4.

206. Johnson WG, Scholl TO, Spychala JR, Buyske S, Stenroos ES, Chen X. Common dihydrofolate reductase 19–base pair deletion allele: a novel risk factor for preterm delivery. Amer J Clin Nutrition. 2005; 81: 664–8.

# *Index*